LANGUAGES AND LINGUISTICS

APHASIA

CLINICAL MANIFESTATIONS, TREATMENT OPTIONS AND IMPACT ON QUALITY OF LIFE

LANGUAGES AND LINGUISTICS

Additional books in this series can be found on Nova's website under the Series tab.

Additional e-books in this series can be found on Nova's website under the e-book tab.

LANGUAGES AND LINGUISTICS

APHASIA

CLINICAL MANIFESTATIONS, TREATMENT OPTIONS AND IMPACT ON QUALITY OF LIFE

CHRISTINA T. ROGERS
EDITOR

New York

Library of Congress Cataloging-in-Publication Data

Names: Rogers, Christina T., editor.
Title: Aphasia : clinical manifestations, treatment options, and impact on quality of life / editor, Christina T. Rogers.
Description: Hauppauge, New York : Nova Science Publishers, [2015] | Series: Languages and linguistics | Includes index.
Identifiers: LCCN 2015038876 | ISBN 9781634839938 (hardcover)
Subjects: LCSH: Aphasia. | Aphasia--Treatment.
Classification: LCC RC425 .A39 2015 | DDC 616.85/52--dc23 LC record available at http://lccn.loc.gov/2015038876

Published by Nova Science Publishers, Inc. † New York

Contents

PREFACE

The loss (complete or partial) of verbal language as a result of some brain condition with preservation of the primary inputs (like auditory, visual or somatosensory projections) and outputs (like motor projections) can be defined as aphasia. The first chapter of this book deals, principally, with some psychological and epistemological issues in the aphasia topic. It discusses the models and approaches for characterizing aphasia. People who develop aphasia must adjust their lifestyles and learn to cope with the activity limitations that follow from their disability. Aphasia can profoundly affect a person's capacity for academic achievement, occupation, social participation, and also financing. This is especially true for children, who have yet to go out into the world to become a member of society. Chapter two and three discuss the phenomenon and impact of acquired aphasia in children. The final chapter examines subcortical aphasia.

Chapter 1 - Aphasia is a neurogenic condition while language is not. In the aphasia field, the direction of reasoning should go from brain injury to verbal impairment; the logical implication is one-way. When the logical implication is inverted, the conclusion is false. This principle allows predicting wrong inferences when the reasoning goes in the reverse order. Maybe that was the cause of the impasse suffered on the matter for more than a century and a half. When prospective approaches are not possible, and trying to attenuate the deficits of retrospective ones, then all the patients should undergo the same psychological evaluations. Post-mortem aphasia studies are always retrospective. Curiously, they are still taken as 'definite'. Aphasia patterns have to be discovered independently of their biological basis in order to avoid circularity; besides, any combination of the latent language impairments has to be recognized. New models concerning the relationship between brain and language have emerged. Beyond the novelty of the instrument used for data collection, deep methodological considerations are necessary not only for discovering the dissociations and interactions among neuropsychological functions, but also for studying the consistency among the different approaches, samples and instruments employed. Nowadays, such consistency has been magnified by dissemination. The impetus to reach consensus with psychological events has led to the shocking situation in which an article published in 1984, for example, has been quoted almost 22,000 times by April of 2015 as synonymous with the procedure for demonstrating diagnosis. Considering the guidelines of 2011 for primary progressive aphasia (PPA) that number was almost 800 in just four years. If the conceptual and the operational definitions are confused, the theory gets into an endless loop. Additionally, the use of typical cases seriously restricts progress. Despite significant improvements observed in the psychological methods during the last years, the psychological outcomes are still puzzling. The 'comprehension-expression' organization and the 'semantics- syntax' one involve two different systems of classification which are not mutually excluding. Unlike the dissociation between comprehension and expression, the dissociation between semantics and syntax is not easy to observe, even using complex linguistic evaluations. Syntax involves relationships among semantic units but, simultaneously, produces a higher-order semantic unit. Researchers evaluate those levels of 'semantic' units to differentiate semantics vs. syntax. The methodology is unclear because changing parts involves changing the whole.

Neuropsychology has two parts. If the validity of the psychological outcomes is doubtful, any language neurobiological model will be doubtful.

Chapter 2 - Acquired Childhood Aphasia (ACA) is a medical phenomenon which is still mostly unknown and often disregarded. One reason for this disregard is the rarity of aphasia in children often being emphasized, and the prognosis being assumed to be more favorable for children and adolescents than for adults. Another common reason for the disregard is the lack of understanding the clinical picture of aphasia in children. The provided chapter offers a broad overview of possible definitions, symptoms, prognosis and outcomes of Acquired Childhood Aphasia and the impact on quality of life for the affected children and adolescents and their families. It goes on to show that the prognosis is not as favorable as often proclaimed, and impacts the affected children and their families in numerous ways. Finally, this chapter points out possibilities of therapeutic intervention and provides examples of measures of support for the families.

Chapter 3 - People who develop aphasia must adjust their lifestyle and learn to cope with the activity limitations that result from their disability. Aphasia can profoundly affect a person's capacity for academic achievement as well as their occupational competency, social participation, and ability to manage finances. This is especially true for young people, who have yet to fully learn how to participate as a member of society. Young people who acquire aphasia are likely to have a poor record at school and have difficulties completing higher education and getting a job. They also might be unable to pass a written test for a driver's license. Young people with aphasia who wish to contribute to the community and be engaged in social activities might not achieve these goals and might feel isolated. In the worst case, they might shut other people out of their lives and withdraw from society. In this chapter, the authors describe the long-term prognosis of three individuals who became aphasic in their childhood or youth and discuss how young people with aphasia can best be rehabilitated.

Chapter 4 - The concept that aphasia is caused by subcortical lesions dates back to the 1970s. However, this subject is still controversial, even today. Many researchers believe that the cortex is the neural center for cognitive functions, including language, and aphasic symptoms observed after subcortical lesions may result, in fact, from functional impairment of cortical activity. In contrast, other authors have advocated a specific role of subcortical structures in language. Advancements in their understanding have resulted in a change of focus for this issue. The term subcortical aphasia encompasses cases of aphasia resulting from lesions located below the cortex, which includes lesions to the basal ganglia, thalamus, and white matter. Advancements in their understanding of the fascicles that travel over the white matter and that connect different cortical areas related to language have revealed that white matter lesions can produce various changes in language. Thus, to elucidate the role of subcortical structures in language, unique injuries to the basal ganglia and thalamus must be separated from those that affect the white matter. The aim of this chapter is to present evidence for the specific involvement of the basal ganglia and thalamus in vocal production, speech, and language. Hypophonia, difficulties in speech initiation, disfluency, syntactic deficits and semantic-lexical disorders are specifically discussed. Thalamic and basal ganglia lesions seem to accompany more complex deficits of language. As the entire cortex has access to subcortical structures, even Broca's and Wernicke's areas, through cortico-subcortical loops, subcortical structures are predominantly integration structures and thus can participate in different aspects of communicative function. The participation of fronto-subcortical circuits and the integration with the posterior cerebral areas has been proposed. Subcortical structures possibly play an important evolutionary role in language acquisition by humans. Basal ganglia and the thalamus may have adapted its own *modus operandi* for speech functions. The cortico-subcortical network and the interrelationship between corticality and subcorticality should be considered to fully comprehend the function of language.

In: Aphasia
Editor: Christina T. Rogers

ISBN: 978-1-63483-993-8

Chapter 1

Models and Approaches for Characterizing Aphasia: Psychological and Epistemological Perspectives

Dr. Nora Silvana Vigliecca*
Consejo Nacional de Investigaciones Científicas y Técnicas de la Argentina (CONICET).
Instituto de Humanidades (IDH). Universidad Nacional de Córdoba, y Servicio de Neurocirugía del Hospital Córdoba, Córdoba, Argentina

Abstract

Aphasia is a neurogenic condition while language is not. In the aphasia field, the direction of reasoning should go from brain injury to verbal impairment; the logical implication is one-way. When the logical implication is inverted, the conclusion is false. This principle allows predicting wrong inferences when the reasoning goes in the reverse order. Maybe that was the cause of the impasse suffered on the matter for more than a century and a half. When prospective approaches are not possible, and trying to attenuate the deficits of retrospective ones, then all the patients should undergo the same psychological evaluations. Post-mortem aphasia studies are always retrospective. Curiously, they are still taken as

* Email: nsvigliecca@gmail.com

'definite'. Aphasia patterns have to be discovered independently of their biological basis in order to avoid circularity; besides, any combination of the latent language impairments has to be recognized. New models concerning the relationship between brain and language have emerged. Beyond the novelty of the instrument used for data collection, deep methodological considerations are necessary not only for discovering the dissociations and interactions among neuropsychological functions, but also for studying the consistency among the different approaches, samples and instruments employed. Nowadays, such consistency has been magnified by dissemination. The impetus to reach consensus with psychological events has led to the shocking situation in which an article published in 1984, for example, has been quoted almost 22,000 times by April of 2015 as synonymous with the procedure for demonstrating diagnosis. Considering the guidelines of 2011 for primary progressive aphasia (PPA) that number was almost 800 in just four years. If the conceptual and the operational definitions are confused, the theory gets into an endless loop. Additionally, the use of typical cases seriously restricts progress. Despite significant improvements observed in the psychological methods during the last years, the psychological outcomes are still puzzling. The 'comprehension-expression' organization and the 'semantics- syntax' one involve two different systems of classification which are not mutually excluding. Unlike the dissociation between comprehension and expression, the dissociation between semantics and syntax is not easy to observe, even using complex linguistic evaluations. Syntax involves relationships among semantic units but, simultaneously, produces a higher-order semantic unit. Researchers evaluate those levels of 'semantic' units to differentiate semantics vs. syntax. The methodology is unclear because changing parts involves changing the whole.

Neuropsychology has two parts. If the validity of the psychological outcomes is doubtful, any language neurobiological model will be doubtful.

Initial Comments

This is an essay which deals, principally, with some psychological and epistemological issues in the aphasia topic. The article has more questions than answers, which is good news. When there are many questions, there is material to work. In contrast, when something is perfect and 'definite' there is nothing to do. Science is perfectible; it needs problems to evolve.

Today, there is so much neurobiological data to process that the core of reasoning tends to be weak. Instead, literature reviews and summaries of hundreds of articles abound. Data from the new technologies along with the demands of overproduction from the current scientific system overwhelm researchers with a lot of information, which is difficult to crystallize in theories. Considering neuropsychological studies in particular, it could be said that, at the moment, there is just one dominant theory for the neurobiological basis of language. The globalization and the international work networks favor consensus and a tendency to fall into absolutisms as a way to compensate, perhaps, for such level of data production. It is as if all the neuropsychological researchers belong to the same laboratory thus leading to share the same theory. Simultaneously, there is a proliferation of concepts, terms, and proposals emerging from other disciplines and interdisciplines (such as the linguistics and its branches, or the neuropsychiatry and its syndrome-specialties) which complicates the panorama.

Concerning some of these concepts and terms, in this work the phonetic-phonological and the pragmatic aspects of communication will not be treated unless otherwise indicated. Although some authors integrate the fields of semantics and pragmatics they will be separated here as much as possible. The concepts of 'context' or 'intentions' may be used to partially replace the broad scope of pragmatics. Besides, only the most formal aspects of natural verbal languages will be discussed and any linguistic unit, such as a word or a sentence, will be considered a 'semantic' unit. Accordingly, a sentence will be defined here as a linguistic (not a grammatical) unit consisting of one [1] or more words that are syntactically 'and' semantically linked to produce a complete thought, i.e., if those words are perfectly organized in their syntactic functions (as determiners, nouns, verbs, etc. throughout the sentence) but they do not produce sentence meaning, then those (empty/ meaningless) words will not form a sentence unit; simultaneously, if the syntactic constructions do not contribute to produce sentence meaning, then those (disorganized) constructions will not form a sentence unit. This was done this way by mainly considering the use (and/or interpretation) of sentences in experimental settings.

Trying to simplify the presentation and/ or avoid the use of many linguistic terms, to the extent that this is possible, some terms will be fused: The lexical and semantic characteristics will be indistinctly seen as part of the same process, being the lexical aspects included in the semantic ones. The same will be done with the morphological and syntactic characteristics, which

[1] Sometimes one single word, which apparently lacks of the conventional structure of a sentence, can transmit the meaning of a whole sentence. In the same way, one single sound can transmit the meaning of a whole word.

will be seen as part of the morphosyntactic process. The present essay attempts to reduce data and names in favor of expressions which involve reasoning, methodology, and inquiring.

This is not a detailed exposition of the models, theories, and approaches that exist for aphasia (and/ or language), but rather a discussion about their underlying method/ epistemology as a whole. The basis for using the terms of semantics and syntax are basically treated with the attempt of stimulating the discussion. A particular viewpoint is all the time present. As well, the value of psychometry in the scope is reconsidered.

INTRODUCTION

The loss (complete or partial) of verbal language as a result of some brain condition with preservation of the primary inputs (like auditory, visual or somatosensory projections) and outputs (like motor projections) can be defined as aphasia.

Sinanović et al. [1] propose a definition which points out the predominantly mixed nature of the condition in its clinical manifestations:

> 'Aphasia is a loss or impairment of verbal communication, which occurs as a consequence of brain dysfunction. It manifests as impairment of almost all verbal abilities, e.g., abnormal verbal expression, difficulties in understanding spoken or written language, repetition, naming, reading and writing.' pp 79.

Regarding primary progressive aphasia (PPA), Mesulam, et al. [2] state:

> 'The diagnosis of primary progressive aphasia (PPA) requires the fulfillment of three core criteria. First, the patient should have an aphasic disorder of recent onset as manifested by distortions of word usage or comprehension that cannot be attributed to more elementary motor or perceptual deficits. Second, this language impairment should constitute the most salient neurobehavioural deficit and the chief impediment to the pursuit of customary daily living activities during the initial stages of the illness. Third, the underlying disease should be neurodegenerative and, therefore, progressive.' pp 1538.

In general, and according to the definitions provided as examples, aphasia is understood as a condition secondary to brain impairment. Naturally, this concept does not extend to the communication system defined as 'language' which, at any rate, is related to brain enhancement and whose socio-educational genesis is beyond dispute.

Although both aphasia and language are neuropsychological processes, aphasia is a neurogenic (pathological) condition while language is not.

Epistemologically speaking, in the field of aphasia the direction of reasoning should always go from brain injury to verbal impairment since the logical implication is one-way. It is well-known that, when the logical implication is inverted, the conclusion is false. This principle allows predicting wrong inferences when the reasoning goes in the reverse order. Maybe this was the cause of the impasse suffered on the matter for more than a century and a half.

Away from logic, the feasibility with which medical studies can be performed cannot be neglected. When aphasia prospective approaches are not possible, and trying to attenuate the deficits of retrospective ones, then all the patients should undergo the same psychological evaluations.[2] Post-mortem aphasia studies are always retrospective. Curiously, they are still taken as 'definite' [3], even if the term 'definite' is incompatible with Science [4].

The (prospective) studies of Tyler and other authors, which are shown next, were selected for their careful experimental designs. This situation allows seeing the variables more clearly and beginning the analysis more comfortably.

Tyler et al. [5] carried out a functional neuroimaging study in which patients with left hemisphere damage or healthy participants listened to spoken sentences that either contained a syntactically ambiguous or matched unambiguous phrase. According to sample selection criteria ('Mini-Mental State Examination' or 'Raven's Colored Progressive Matrices') [3] none of the patients were cognitively impaired. Regarding the experimental spoken sentences, those authors stated: 'Even though the ambiguous phrases were presented in a neutral context, subjects have preferences for one syntactic interpretation over another, which affect the ease with which ambiguities can be resolved (Rayner and Duffy, 1986)'. This preference situation, which Rayner and Duffy [6] define as lexical ambiguity, was then controlled by the

[2] It has to be clear that undergoing the same psychological evaluations is different from achieving (or intentionally searching) the same result patterns for all the patients.

[3] Raven Matrices and Mini-Mental are not equivalent tests of cognitive performance; besides since the Mini-Mental is a predominantly verbal test, it is sensitive to left hemisphere lesions [9]. It would be interesting to see the correlation between the tests selected to include patients (as dependent variables) and the results of the experiment.

authors through the incorporation, in the experimental design, of the dominant/preferred and subordinate/non-preferred conditions as independent variables. Interestingly, that was the situation which produced brain-functioning differences between patients with left hemisphere damage and healthy participants in the ambiguous phrases. Beyond neurobiological findings, patients were insensitive to those preferences, and that situation was taken (based on other control tasks) as an index of syntactic rather than semantic deficits. This is an example where researchers evaluate two levels of semantic units (the preferred and non-preferred sentences based on the content of a previous clause) to intentionally differentiate syntax from semantics, i.e., rooted in two semantic categories, researchers get to different 'syntactic' categories thus not only assuming that syntax is, in this experimental context, different from semantics but also concluding that it was syntax (and not semantics) which caused the observed deficits. The form of the verb (either 'is' or 'are') was the cue which these authors used to convert an initially semantic context in a syntactic one. The patients recruited in such work showed almost no semantic impairments compared with syntactic ones (0-6% vs. 0-47%, respectively) in a sentence-picture matching test. This result was also used for interpretations.

Tyler and Marslen-Wilson [7] had previously observed that syntactic decisions are affected by prior semantic context, and that syntactic processing is not autonomous from semantics; i.e., the syntactic structure of a sentence is computed with reference to its meaning. Marslen-Wilson and Tyler [8] had also observed that 'lexical, structural (syntactic), and interpretative knowledge sources communicate and interact during processing in an optimally efficient and accurate manner.'

Some Epistemological Commentaries about Semantics and Syntax: From Psychological Interaction to Neurobiological Dissociation

Independently of the works quoted above, it is well-known that when the interaction between two or more factors has been verified, it cannot be concluded that only one of those factors is causing the studied effects. As well, when two or more attributes (factors/ variables) with their corresponding categories and/or levels of assessment are confused, it cannot be inferred that any of those attributes explains the phenomenon under study.

For example, and going well away from the language subject, if chocolate cake mixtures are put into small molds and vanilla cake mixtures are put into large molds, then it cannot be inferred that either the small molds or the chocolate mixtures produce, let's say, the most attractive cakes. That is so because the effect of chocolate cake mixtures combined with large molds, and the effect of vanilla cake mixtures combined with small molds are missing.[4] Although the cake needs from both attributes (mixtures and molds) to be produced, the process involved between the initial attributes and their final fusion is not trivial, represents the method, and is also irreversible. In this case, the attributes of cake mixtures and molds are essentially different in their quality, and the two attributes want to be related. So, and in order to be sure of the causes and effects of such relationship, the levels or categories for the mixtures, and the levels or categories for the molds have to be clearly distinguished and combined.[5] If qualities and levels are confused (without clearly identifying the types of variables and their categories) as in the example of the cakes, it will be impossible to know what it is measured and interpreted.

Going back to the language topic, the fact that a 'perfect' sentence activates certain brain areas, whereas an 'imperfect' (or more difficult to perceive) sentence activates other brain areas, does not necessarily validate, let's say, the semantics-syntax neuropsychological model (see below the hegemonic neuropsychological model) because it is not clear if the qualities and levels of the two supposedly assessed attributes have been well distinguished.[6] Using one polysemantic word in different linguistic contexts is

---

[4] Other examples of levels or categories for the mixtures can be: 'without sugar', 'with a little of sugar', and 'with a lot of sugar'; whereas, for the molds, they can be: 'square', 'triangle', and 'circle'. Maybe one variable only has qualities while the other variable only has levels to be assessed. The problem is not the type of the selected variables (qualitative or quantitative) but the confusion among the categories or levels of their measures. Such confusion tends to obscure the variables' effects.

[5] Apart from the researchers, who represent the designers of the method, there are the interviewees who represent the receivers of the final product. If the qualities and levels of the initial attributes and their assessments are not clearly distinguished, the researcher's viewpoint may be confused with the interviewee's viewpoint. The problem is that the final product resulting from the interaction between molds and mixtures also has attributes or variables, such as the different shapes and flavors of the cakes. But such assessments have to be differentiated from the assessments of the initial materials, such as the shapes and flavors of the molds and mixtures. On the other hand, it is possible that researchers (or their techniques) are seeing how the interviewees are cutting the cake rather than seeing how the interviewees are appreciating or savoring the cake.

[6] Although verbal neuropsychological events are so much complex than cakes and molds, the following equivalence can be posed: The contrast between some correct verbal meaning (e.g., the meaning of a word) put into a perfect sentence versus some ambiguous verbal

not simple to experimentally distinguish and match, particularly for semantics and syntax, which are two interacting and highly complex psychological functions. Researchers are changing two categories at a time (one part and the whole), for two intricate attributes which, still, may differ in their quality. Even supposing that exactly one single detail was changed for otherwise identical sentences, maybe the studied brain is distinguishing something different from what is interpreted by researchers. For example, maybe the brain is distinguishing different types of 'semantic structures' (such as the meaning of the sentence as a whole versus the meanings of single words or fragmented sentential subunits) instead of different types of 'syntactic structures'. Beyond semantics and syntax, maybe the brain is distinguishing the linguistic structure which is more attractive, consolidated, usual, easy to decipher, and/ or singular than the other.

Syntax involves relationships among semantic units but, simultaneously, produces a higher-order semantic unit. Interestingly, some researchers evaluate those levels of 'semantic' units (e.g., words or sentences) to differentiate semantics vs. syntax, being the sentence level reserved for syntax.

When the method is not clear, results can be freely interpreted with the theory at hand. The problem in this scope in particular is that there are many linguistic theories (for reviews see, [10-15]) but very few neurobiological ones [16-18] to interpret neuropsychological issues.

Nowadays, and psychologically speaking, researchers tend to put in the center of experimental analyses to semantic and syntactic processes, with a clear preference towards studying these processes with comprehensive tasks [16-17].[7] Neurobiologically speaking, and certainly influenced by the theory of the dorsal and ventral streams for language [19] (including its inspirational theory for visual perception [20, see also 21]) the anatomical dorsal and ventral pathways have now become the main neurobiological explanation for semantics and syntax. Curiously, the original work for the dual stream [19] was predominantly based on speech perception and speech production rather than on semantics and syntax. Beyond the current inclusion of pragmatics as a neurobiological subject of interest, and the discovering of new brain centers and pathways for language processing [16-18], the fact is that semantics and

meaning put into an imperfect sentence would be similar to the contrast between chocolate cake mixtures put into small molds versus vanilla cake mixtures put into large molds. The same would apply to some correct/ ordered morphosyntactic construction versus some ambiguous/ disordered morphosyntactic one. The methodology is unclear because, in this case, changing some parts involves changing the whole.

[7] There is also a preference towards studying the syntactic process, which seems to be clearer than semantics for measuring and interpreting (see below).

syntax are considered essential (and comparable) linguistic categories under this view: Today, the hegemonic neuropsychological model for language is represented by this view.

At this point, some questions can be asked: Has morphosyntax a different quality than semantics? If this is not true (and they have the same quality): Does morphosyntax involve a different level of analysis (either inferior or superior) than semantics? If this is true, and assuming that researchers have to be located in the superior level to analyze the inferior one: Is morphosyntax an inferior level of analysis within semantics? Or is semantics an inferior level of analysis within morphosyntax?

If semantics and syntax differ in their quality, they cannot be compared in the same way that 'cake mixtures' and 'molds' cannot be compared. They cannot be directly assessed as subsets belonging to the same category and/or be measured by the same yardstick. If some relationship between semantics and syntax wants to be established with reference to another variable, they will need more complex analyses, than those of the cake example, to avoid psychological confusion between qualities and levels.

Maybe semantics (in its broadest sense) is not a level in the hierarchy of verbal language, as are commonly considered the phonetic-phonological and the morphosyntactic ones. Perhaps it is more an attribute which breaks through the levels of other verbal attributes, thus acting all the time as a parallel (or surrounding) process rather than as a sequential one.

Syntax involves the rules for articulation/ linking, which are easy to teach and learn, but the rules for understanding are more difficult to find and transmit. (Perhaps this is due to the fact that syntactic rules are more stable and restricted, while semantic rules are more chaotic and versatile).

Usually, semantics and syntax are seen as complementary processes where semantics would be the content/ the gnosia/ the 'what' while syntax/ morphosyntax would be the form/ the praxia/ the 'how' (or where). However, and without forgetting that verbal language is a biosocial instrument developed by human beings to better control and organize communication, the following analogy can be proposed: By considering semantics as the content of 'water' and morphosyntax as the human tools or 'containers' which gives form to such content, water will not stop being water by taking the shape of the containers that human beings invented to contain, control, organize and understand it. On the contrary, if the containers disappear when human beings have already become accustomed to the containers, the water will slip through their fingers and an important part of human beings will be lost, i.e., as human beings can no longer manipulate water, they will enter into crisis. [8] The analogy is used to show not only the importance of tools for humans, but also (and for didactic issues) the relative importance that contents and containers may have in certain contexts.

Considering morphosyntax just as a tool, semantics would not only represent the content 'poured into/ passed through' the morphosyntactic structure but also 'the root and the goal' of the process mediated by syntactic sequencing. Surrounded by this wide-ranging structure or matrix, morphosyntax would be an inferior level of analysis within semantics. As it will be seen below, this perspective is apparently difficult to conceive or understand by the hegemonic neuropsychological model for language. Such misunderstanding may lead to interpret results in the most convenient way or, most probably, in the easiest way to be carried out or decoded. Such way is usually the linear and analytic one. The problem is that interpretations generate theories.

The attempt of analyzing the complex interactions between semantics and syntax by taking into account just one epistemological point of view (e.g., the linear or the nonlinear one) may lead to a reductionism which can detract the whole process of verbal processing in any direction. Returning to the example of the contents and containers, the attempt of reducing the complexity of semantics to simplistic (linear and partial) syntactic analyses would be equivalent to try to understand the essence of a cake by seeing the details of the mold. The analysis in the opposite direction can be proposed as follows: the attempt of expanding/ observing the particularities of syntactic analysis through a more comprehensive semantic view would be equivalent to try to understand the details of the molds by seeing all the ingredients of the cake mixtures. Although both expressions are strange, the second is not so unrealistic in the sense that a mold has turned out a useful instrument, created to improve the presentation of the cake, but not vice versa.

Catani and Bambini [16] propose a theoretical model for analyzing social communication and language in which five levels are hierarchically and serially organized according to developmental and evolutionary aspects. When describing the level 3, which is the 'anterior temporal networks for lexical and

[8] Usually, when human beings become accustomed to a new tool, it is difficult to go back to an old one. This can lead to confound the adjectives of 'new', 'later', or even 'human', with 'better' or 'superior'. Taking into account the specific context in which scientists have to work, the experimental method is also a human (logical) tool, necessary in scientific settings, but it cannot be compared with the old, wild, and wise intuition, which human beings are progressively losing. Maybe syntax is closer to the experimental method (thus favoring syntax study) while semantics is closer to intuition.

semantic processing', the authors state: '...the temporal cortex is involved in selecting verbal labels for objects in a posterior–anterior progression of word comprehension, from generic to specific levels of precision.' When describing the level 4, which is the 'fronto-temporal network for syntactic analysis', for some reason the authors intentionally use the term 'analysis'. Although they say that the Wernicke's region participates in syntactic analysis, they do not specify a certain direction for either the progression or the level of precision as they did for the level 3. They affirm: 'successful syntactic processing requires the interplay between lexical properties and syntactic analysis, which is mediated by the joint activation of the whole frontotemporal system connected through the long segment of the arcuate fasciculus.'

It is not clear whether the term 'syntactic analysis' was used by Catani and Bambini [16] as synonymous with 'syntactic processing' or if it was used as a singular way of conceiving (or studying) the particularities of syntactic processing. Besides, at first sight, both processes seem to be analytic. If that is so, not only the semantic processing would go from something more generic to something more specific but also the syntactic processing.

To understand the model of Catani and Bambini [16] some alternative appreciations can be formulated concerning semantics and syntax. While continuing the discussion of the differences and interactions between those two functions, conciliations among terms or concepts will be searched.

Compared with syntax, maybe semantics is a more complex process that surely exceeds verbal language and human scope, as well as partial and linear analyses; it is probably more related to the principles of holistic perception or even to the gestalt theory, and it cannot be understood outside its context or background, at all ages. In the attempt to find a schematic representation for this process, semantics could imaginatively be seen as a network of meaningful contents or symbols, which mostly are intersecting with each other; some may be closer to others, some may be stronger than others, and some may be isolated from others. The patterns of their relationships would be dynamically determined, among other reasons, according to the standards, points of view, needs, and the significance for survival of the people involved in communication. Those patterns not only would be transversally affected by human interaction, at the very moment of communication, but also longitudinally, throughout each step of the development. Considering that verbal labels are human conventions established for certain meanings, the association between the original network of nonverbal contents and the verbal construction of linked labels is probably the main characteristic of semantic integration. Therefore, the convergences and divergences between phonological and morphosyntactic features will also affect the patterns of semantic relationships.

If all the possible linked labels are visualized as a nonlinear surface, and a sentence as a curve line, a dynamic interaction can be conceived where the movements around a certain meaning, or the constructions around a certain sentence, will have more or less significance. Accordingly, the movements and constructions will act at different moments (initially, subsequently, or simultaneously) depending on the context. Movements, constructions, and moments are linguistic associations acting in a certain context. But if only one association is considered the most significant, and the other associations are considered just pieces of the first association, there will be an oversimplification of the whole process. For current neurobiological theories, syntax seems to excel semantics as a superior level: as a more abstract representation, higher- order function, and later-in-time stage. However, it is highly probable that both linguistic functions require complementary forces interacting with each other, as part of the same process. Considering the history of linguistic knowledge, it is difficult to explain why the isolated line of a sentence (just a handful of linked labels) became more important than its surrounding matrix. Maybe that was so because the final expression of verbal language follows a linear arrangement, which is a necessary (but not sufficient) characteristic in this type of communication.

Bearing in mind the need of interaction between semantics and syntax, it can be observed that sometimes 'pure' thoughts go faster than words, thus producing incorrect utterances. However, when the semantic associations are harmonious with the morphosyntactic ones, utterances will go out correctly aligned. In order to convert 'pure' thoughts in 'verbal' thoughts and, then, in explicit utterances, everything that takes place simultaneously and involving many areas and functions of the brain (such as attention, perception, gnosia, praxia, memory, associations of any type, social-emotional adjustment, global cognition, and so on) at some point has to follow the linear mode of verbal language.[9] Some of the associations that the brain can do to semantically organize an utterance can be deduced from the nature of the errors committed during spontaneous speech: The presence of paraphasias of any type, the inopportune influence of emotional sources, as well as the previous and

[9] When thoughts go out correctly aligned through the final verbal and linear mode, it is not difficult to imagine the similarity with different containers passing through an assembly line, in which the different contents are correctly placed in their specific containers.

subsequent thoughts, which can be jumbled up with the current expression, are frequent examples of these associations.[10]

When the syntactic analysis of a sentence is defined as a sort of a formal reasoning, maybe such reasoning is conceived like a sequence of (empty) compartments useful to organize the world of word labels, which would follow a similar organization to the world of nonverbal representations.

Verbal ability requires that all that internal universe of feelings and ideas finally goes out aligned and synthesized for that narrow channel of morphosyntactic 'molds'. In that channel, every part of every linguistic unit has to be assembled with the next in order to be converted in a meaningful and well-organized expression.[11] Maybe for this reason expression (speech production) is sometimes confused with syntax. However, comprehension (speech perception) also requires that the received message pass through that narrow channel: All the received contents must be correctly placed in their specific morphosyntactic 'molds' so that the receptor's brain could deal with a well-organized/ decodable verbal unit; i.e., all the words and/ or sounds of the message have to be ordered in such a linear mode because, otherwise, the message will not be perceived as a verbal one. Afterwards, the verbal message would semantically spread to the whole brain thus reaching the different networks of memory and cognition for a whole and multimodal interpretation.

Semantics would be dynamically guided by an advanced organization established during the phylogeny and ontogeny that resembles the process of perception: A top-down perspective which goes from generic to specific levels of precision (see Catani and Bambini, [16]) would be dominant. Under this organization, it is necessary to first recognize the general meaning (the whole background) to then analyze/ select a specific meaning or detail.

Taking into account some of the variables usually studied in the laboratory, the linguistic preferences [5], levels of difficulty, and frequencies of use, which by the way are all interconnected, are probably more related to semantics than to syntax.

Within the cultural factors associated to both linguistic processes, morphosyntactic knowledge would be more compulsorily taught, and more sociologically and logically organized, while semantic knowledge would be

---

[10] Probably this kind of errors affects communication more seriously than the 'purely syntactic ones' (see below). To what extend such more serious semantic errors are produced because the syntactic compartments have been seriously broken is an open question.

[11] 'There is a lack of consensus on the nature of the process of linking; that is, how the conceptual form of thoughts determines the form of the spoken expressions used to describe them' [15].

more intuitively perceived and more automatically and biologically organized, to a certain extent. Usually, it is easier to show or share semantics than to explain it. Maybe for this reason it is more difficult for neurobiological researchers to operationalize and analyze semantics components than syntactic ones. Probably, the more human is an attribute, the easier is to analyze it. Reciprocally (and paradoxically for humans), the more primitive is an attribute, the easier is to integrate and perceive it. The semantic ability involved in extracting the figure (the most relevant meaning) from a background of competing linguistic stimuli, according to internal and external demands, is dynamically and progressively constructed along with the rest of the cognitive abilities. With time, and living in a coherent world, human beings will learn to prefer the meaningful stimuli and reject the meaningless ones according to: their frequency and quality of appearance, consistency to reward, usefulness to find biological or social solutions, pertinence for a certain situation, etc. Verbal stimuli are not the exception.

To have an idea of the complexity of semantic processing even using single-word tasks, or just two prepositions, see Wright, et al. [22] as well as Marslen-Wilson and Tyler [8] for an experimental approach which uses picture naming and word–picture matching; see also Kelleher and van Genabith [23], for a computational model which uses two prepositions and shows nonlinear images.

When sentence semantic processing wants to be assessed in functional neuroimaging studies, a common way that researchers use to produce a modification which affects the meaning of a sentence (without changing syntax) is to change a single word in the sentence. This procedure is enough to reach the desired effect with clear experimental conditions: Changing several words, using implausible sentences or series of unconnected words, involve more variables and complicate interpretations. But changing just one single word (with high linguistic weight) may be semantically equivalent to change the entire sentence. Considering an example of Newman, et al. [24] (also quoted by Hagoort and Indefrey, [17] and by Murphy [15]): ‘my mother ironed a kiss’; the misuse (unusual presentation) of a single word changes the meaning of the whole sentence. Since the highest semantic level of the sentence unit is dominant, all the lower-level semantic units will cooperate to form the biggest conceptual representation (or the most relevant perception), no matter if the generated image/ meaning is usual or unusual. So, it is highly probable that, for the receptor's brain, 'the meaning of each linguistic unit and the global meaning of the sentence are determined simultaneously' [25].[12]

On the contrary, the change of a single morphosyntactic sub-unit or detail does not change that easy the perception of the whole meaning of the sentence. Actually, it can be observed that, in the spontaneous/ colloquial speech of healthy people, a lot of morphosyntactic errors are committed without affecting communication. By using the same example quoted above, the change of the word 'ironed' by 'give' instead of 'gave' or 'gives' (i.e., 'my mother give a kiss') maintains the meaning of the new sentence in general terms. By using another example with a more serious error like 'the park was placed on the statue' (an inversion error which can be mediated by semantic or syntactic reasons) listeners will still understand the entire meaning of the sentence. That is so because listeners correct the unfeasible/ funny detail thus maintaining the balance between the whole and the parts [26]. When this balance in the sentence is broken, and the whole meaning succumbs to the parts, the sentence becomes fragmented: Verbal language disintegration occurs when the context, the subjective and objective cues, as well as the communication efforts made by the involved persons are useless.[13]

Beyond specific cases of verbal language fragmentation, researchers try to maintain the balance between the whole and the parts by modifying just a semantic or syntactic detail in the experimental condition and leaving constant the rest. In this attempt, and beyond the interaction between semantics and syntax, researchers also involve the interaction between analysis and synthesis, which is dependent of age and education among other factors. Complex tasks involving these four functions are better accomplished from teenage years onwards. Complementary cognitive requirements such as divided attention, mental tracking, attention span, working memory, and executive functions may be necessary for these tasks. For example, it is well-known that if an analytic task wants to be carried out, the interviewee first has to have an idea of what is going to be divided. So, if the background of the biggest stimulus cannot be preserved by any cause, the analytic task will be impossible to be carried out. These developmental aspects are not ignored by researchers.

[12] Unlike the semantic processing of a sentence, the syntactic processing probably involves that each linguistic subunit and the global syntactic structure are determined consecutively, particularly in experimental contexts (see below).

[13] When the language fragmentation goes beyond a single sentence or moment, and affects the entire verbal language, it is time to analyze the type and level of distortion in order to determine the type and level of aphasia.

Complex syntactic analyses are acquired later in the development. Furthermore, when this learning is incipient, it is probable that the more conscious and broken is the syntactic analysis, the more difficult is its intuitive perception: Children probably have to inhibit synthesis or integration in order to analyze. Later, they will automatically complement analysis and synthesis and use them together thus organizing harmonically the sub-units within the biggest unit. Correctness (culture) also depends on the level of education, which is not a minor detail in the neurobiology of language.

Nonverbal processing comes first in the evolution [27, 28], then the verbal-auditory one, and then the verbal-visual one. Concurrently, and as it is reported by Catani and Bambini [16], semantic processing would come first than syntactic analysis. The last acquisitions are the most culturally biased [29] and, usually, the less cognitively crystallized. Brauer, et al. [30], observed that seven-year-old children possess a brain connectivity pattern of the dorsal language route that is similar to the one observed for adults. Those authors affirm: ‘It is at around this age that children start to successfully process more complex and also passive sentence structures’ It is also hypothesized that seven-year-old children do not have yet the ability to process complex sentence structures (as may be processed by adults) since the dorsal pathway is still not yet fully mature. Brauer, et al. [30] also leave open the question about how the connection between neural and syntactic developments actually occurs. In any case, the ability to consciously disentangle the components and rules of syntax in a sentence is a late acquisition.

If syntax was developed to favor the organization and sense of communication (i.e., if the main point of the sentence compartmentalization and word sequencing is to transmit information with meaning) maybe the most important syntactic components are those which are more prone to affect the highest-order meaning. In the erroneous example quoted above (i.e., ‘my mother give a kiss’) the syntactic distortion does not change the meaning of the sentence because, probably, this is a minor detail for communication. To a certain extent it seems that evolution (unlike some researchers) prioritizes meaning over specific details of form and syntax. When morphosyntactic rules are momentarily broken, semantics becomes dominant in order to protect communication: Given a certain conversation in which the speaker cannot articulate sounds or words for an instant, it is common that the speaker claims: "You know what I'm saying;" and it is also common that the listener pay attention to what the speaker wants to say as well as to what he/ she as a listener wants to listen in order to not to interrupt the feedback.

When morphosyntactic resources are at risk, semantic units of any size cannot be constructed or correctly linked with other units. But when semantic resources are at risk, the morphosyntactic resources lose their reason for being; therefore, communication in itself is at risk. However, and contrasting with other types of language, 'pure' verbal language requires from the interaction between semantics and syntax.

Unlike semantics, the syntactic processing described by Catani and Bambini [16] as 'syntactic analysis' is probably more related to the principles of an analytic approach for understanding (or perceiving). Under this perspective, maybe a sentence is conceived as a linear arrangement easily dissectible throughout several compartments, from the beginning to the end of the linguistic unit. When the direct comprehension of a sentence from the beginning to the end (or from the left to the right in the case of reading) is experimentally hampered by a linear configurational complication, such complication is usually defined as a syntactic manipulation in neurobiological research settings. Under the influence of such complication, the sentence linear arrangement has to be altered in its standard form of being perceived (including loops and prolongations), or in its natural way of being explored (including interruptions and comebacks) so that the comprehension task (i.e., the cognitive synthesis or semantic integration) can finally be achieved.[14]

When the syntactic processing is neurobiologically evaluated, there are at least two sentences to be compared being one of them simpler (to be constructed or understood) than the other.[15] When syntactic comprehension and expression are evaluated, researchers may force interviewees to pay attention, for example, to the analysis of the form in which the interviewer is expressing the sentence. By this means, researchers (rather than interviewees) are sometimes putting syntax as figure and semantics as ground.[16] Perhaps the

---

[14] From a simplistic point of view, and excluding complex interactions among semantics, syntax, analysis, and synthesis (see above), it could be said that, overall, when morphosyntactic processing is involved in expression, a top-down arrangement would be dominant; on the contrary when morphosyntactic processing is involved in comprehension, a bottom-up arrangement would be dominant. When the research involves healthy adults and complex syntactic analyses, bottom-up and top-down perspectives will interact.

[15] If math performance is compared to syntactic performance, the operations of 3+3 and 18/3 produce the same result, which might be considered the final meaning, but both operations differ in quality and complexity. Both operations also have their own meanings and labels.

[16] The 10-item version of the Northwestern Anagram Test, used by Catani et al. [31] which measures object- and subject-extracted 'who' questions (e.g., Who is the groom carrying?, Who is carrying the bride?, respectively) apparently is an example. In this test of grammatical processing, which has to be answered with visual stimuli, the patient is asked to order single words, each printed on a separate card, to correctly depict the action in a target picture.

ability to bring awareness to certain unconscious processes (which at the moment of the evaluation are already automatically made) is easier for syntactic than for semantic integration tasks.

Apparently, syntactic manipulations have had positive results for neurobiological findings.

Hagoort and Indefrey [17] observe that sentences containing a subject - relative clause (e.g., "The reporter who attacked the senator admitted the error") are found to be easier to understand than sentences with an object - relative clause (e.g., "The reporter who the senator attacked admitted the error." On the one hand, these authors highlight the integration between semantics and syntax and some subtle questions concerning the impossibility of studying both processes as separated ones are suggested in the introduction of their work. These authors affirm that the degree of separation between networks for syntactic and semantic integration is not so clear:

> "Separation of these networks is nontrivial because syntactic differences are not without semantic consequences…A difference in syntactic structure clearly has immediate consequences for mapping grammatical roles (subject, object) onto thematic roles (agent, undergoer) and hence for the…conceptual/ semantic representation of the sentence" pp 350.

On the other hand, these authors attempt to segregate the two types of processes as much as possible using data from a meta-analysis of numerous functional imaging studies. With this vision in mind, they follow their dissertation writing a subtitle where the syntactic processing is put against the semantic one, and begin such section with this sentence: 'So far, the available information is most clear for the areas involved in syntactic analysis'.

It is beyond any dispute that fertile information can be obtained from the use of some syntactic-analytic paradigms. For example, some interesting effects can be discovered by restricting the syntactic analysis just to comprehension (listening or reading), and by assuming that, before integrating the sentence components as a whole, interviewees can sequentially detect the complication, i.e., interviewees can pay attention to the ambiguity, the error, the difficulty, the object or subject used in a certain order, the verb used in a certain form, etc. when such complications appear in the line of the sentence. Within this framework, Malaia and Newman [32] carried out an EEG study in which they analyzed the topographical distribution of alpha power to identify the time course of the linguistic binding process during word-by-word sentence reading. By manipulating semantic information (e.g., noun animacy) and syntactically-relevant information (e.g., verbal template), these authors demonstrated 'that the processing of semantic and syntactic features during sentence comprehension proceeds in highly integrated fashion using gating of attentional resources to facilitate rapid comprehension, with attentional suppression of global alpha power to facilitate interaction of local networks.'

At the present time, there are few studies which escape from the hegemonic position and, thus, few authors who demonstrate a neurobiological interaction rather than dissociation between semantics and syntax. Besides, and by following the new trend, it is generally assumed that semantics is an inferior level of analysis within morphosyntax: Changes in syntactic structures would not affect semantics or, if so, they can still be considered pure syntactic changes. Under this analytic/ syntactic-dominant view, semantics would apparently be represented by the elementary or lower-level units useful to construct the bigger structure of 'syntax' (not the bigger structure of semantics).

Hagoort and Indefrey [17] affirm that syntactic integration cannot simply be reduced to semantic one. So, and based on neurobiological findings, this trend would include the more basic semantic elements (usually single words or simpler-than-sentence semantic units) within wide-ranging syntactic operations. From this perspective two expressions can be syntactically matched even if they are semantically empty (see, e.g., [5, 8]) but not vice versa. Under this view, syntax is considered superior to semantics, which serves to build syntax.[17]

Linguistic Manipulations and Concepts: Neuropsychological Uses and Interpretations

Disordering or changing the words of a sentence is effortless in view of its linear characteristics; the question is how the interviewee will semantically perceive those changes. Without the researchers' interventions, it is usual that the interviewee's brain correct the input distortions to a great extent. Let's take the following example with five specific words ('car', 'speedy', 'the', 'is', and 'red'), used with an unusual syntactic structure: article + adjective + adjective + verb + noun. Then (and obviously presented in a methodologically reliable

[17] Under this view, the content (e.g., the cake mixture) has turned out useful to improve the presentation of the mold or, worse, the content has turned out to be just as an accessory that can be used or not.

context)[18] it could be possible that a rare expression like 'the red speedy is car' is neurobiologically perceived by the interviewee as a more common sentence like 'the red car is speedy' or 'the speedy car is red'. Thus, the interviewee would be semantically matching (perceptively correcting) the rare expression with a more frequent one. Outside the laboratory, this is a common situation in particular if the wrong sentence is quickly said within a correct linguistic background or context. Even inside the laboratory, the experimental context in which a distortion (or peculiarity) is included is also important: If one unusual sentence is included within a context of usual series of sentences, the change will be easily detected. The balance between usual and unusual conditions is an intervening variable. At once, if one distorted word with low semantic or syntactic weight in the sentence is included within a context of words with high linguistic weight, the change will be uneasily detected. If this is not so, at least it would be worth studying at what time the experimentally manipulated 'sentences' begin to be neurobiologically perceived as fragmented sentences, isolated phrases, or series of words. On the other hand, if semantics wants to be excluded (or preserved constant) from a syntactic experiment, ideally the stimuli to be compared should be equally easy to understand.[19] Besides, in the paradigms that compare sentential conditions in common with non-sentential/ asyntactic ones, these conditions should match in semantics as much as possible, in particular if they are used for making semantic inferences. However, all these control conditions taken together are very difficult to achieve.

In fact, and based on the neurobiological consequences of the current hegemonic theory, it does not matter if semantics and syntax differ in quality or not; they can actually be compared, measured by the same yardstick, and put in the same line of methodological and linguistic analysis. If there is some kind of interaction in their psychological/ initial factors, they finally get dissociated to the searched endpoint. May be this is a case where the end justifies the means because, by these means, researchers have found the

[18] If the expression 'the red speedy is: car' is applied in a context where the interviewees have to guess what moves at high speed, the example will not be relevant. By the way this (personal) semantic association shows how the brain is always looking for a meaning where an unusual expression can fit: A visual image appears, for an unusual expression.

[19] The use of active and passive voice, e.g., is considered a classical paradigm for assessing syntactic processing [5]. However, the level of difficulty and the frequency of use of the two sentences are not matched; passive voice is acquired later and is more difficult to be constructed and understood than active voice. So, not only two levels of syntactic functioning (and two stages of verbal development) are compared, but also two types of semantic units. As said above, researchers are changing two categories at a time for assessing one attribute which includes the other.

neurobiological differences they were looking for. Following this way of thinking it could be said that, at the present time, behavior appears as a sort of 'black box' within the manipulable inputs and dissociable outputs of neurobiological experiments. That is so, even when the inputs in themselves are confused and, also, part of the 'behavioral black box'. Besides, it is difficult to understand that clear outputs can emerge from confused inputs. Hagoort and Indefrey [17] observed, for example, that Brodmann area (BA) 44 activation is clearly driven more strongly by syntactic than by semantic demands, suggesting that this region contains neuronal populations involved in syntactic operations *per se* or that the semantic consequences of such syntactic demands (e.g., difficulty of thematic role assignment) are processed by neuronal populations that differ from those processing other kinds of semantic consequences. [20] This statement leaves open the possibility for other interpretations (more integrative ones) regarding the relevance of semantics compared with syntax. For example, that semantics can only be 'affected' by syntax in the same way that can be affected by many other verbal (and nonverbal) factors or, maybe, that 'semantic integration cannot simply be reduced to syntactic integration' (see above the opposite affirmation expressed by Hagoort and Indefrey, [17]).[21] Almost certainly, verbal integration cannot be reduced to just these two psychological functions, whatever are their natures or levels in the hierarchy of language.

Semantics and syntax can be considered verbal organizers with different rules of organization. Semantics and syntax supposedly represent useful processes to sort, dissociate, and combine words within a linguistic context. It is generally accepted that sorting words by their relationship with the objects

[20] Hagoort and Indefrey [17] also observed a distinctive activation pattern in the posterior left inferior frontal gyrus (LIFG): Syntactic demands activated more dorsal parts (BA 44/45) and semantic demands activated more ventral parts (BA 45/47) across all kinds of increased processing demands (violations, ambiguity, complexity) and in studies performing direct comparisons of high syntactic and semantic processing demands. Additionally, the dorsal/ventral gradient observed in the LIFG seems to be mirrored in the left posterior temporal lobe. Alternatively, Catani and Bambini [16] propose that the fronto-temporal networks for syntactic analysis are associated with the long segment of the arcuate fasciculus (the dorsal network) while the anterior temporal networks for lexical and semantic processing are associated with the middle and inferior longitudinal fasciculus, the uncinate fasciculus, and with the extreme capsule/inferior fronto-occipital fasciculus (the ventral networks). Both teams found dorsal-ventral dissociations for syntactic-semantic operations, respectively, in agreement with the anatomical proposal of Hickok & Poeppel [19].

[21] Actually, the exact words of Hagoort and Indefrey [17]) were: 'syntactic unification cannot simply be reduced to semantic unification.' The term 'unification' is used by these authors to indicate the real-time assembly of the pieces retrieved from memory into larger structures, with contributions from context.

in the world involves a semantically driven process, while sorting words by their relationship with other words in the sentence involves a syntactically driven one. But there is also a world of words, in which every label and group of linked labels not only have their own meanings, but also generate new meanings when they are dissociated or combined. Researchers are trying to elucidate this organization and its rules. However, the hierarchy which organizes the different levels (or categories) of these linguistic processes is still today difficult to validate. I.e., the art of combining elements is cognitively superior to the elements themselves, the problem is that, for verbal language, there is much debate about the art and the elements. Such art is these days interpreted as syntax. However, the combination of elements arises from (and is addressed for) something, which gives sense to the whole creative process. The ability to give sense is semantics. Most probably, multiple psychological functions and sub-functions (including semantics and syntax) are acting together for verbal integration thus involving many connections in many directions in the brain. For example, the generation and preservation of the highest levels of cognition supposedly facilitate the processing of the lowest ones but, for that, the lowest ones have to exist [26]. However, the current (widespread) neuropsychological techniques have not yet transferred such hierarchical integration to statistically based theoretical frameworks.

> 'The notion of bio-physiological dimensions for verbal language (and aphasia) involves the notion of neuropsychological functions and the need of validation... It is a common expression to say that a test measures certain neuropsychological functions. Yet, those functions are concepts which need to be empirically validated...The constructs of verbal comprehension and verbal expression are among the most widely used in literature ...Impairments in such domains may be related to comprehensive and expressive aphasias' [29].

Considering some of the most used neuropsychological constructs in the scope, it is worth noting that semantics and syntax are more abstract concepts than comprehension and expression, which involve a more direct link between their conceptual and empirical definitions. Semantics and syntax, on the other hand, need further studies on the interaction with other verbal and cognitive constructs. The study of the interaction between the semantics-syntax system and other functions such as speech, repetition, naming, reading, writing, phonemic processing, attention, memory, and praxia, among other functions, is essential for both language and aphasia.

Within the field of aphasia, and by using the categories of nonfluent/agrammatic, semantic, and logopenic aphasias, the guidelines proposed for the PPA variants [3] rely more on the semantics-syntax organization than on the comprehension-expression one. Recent empirical studies on the matter [33], however, tend to dichotomize the PPA outcomes towards the classical difference between fluent and nonfluent aphasias, instead of the three variants initially proposed by the guidelines of 2011 [3].

Before continuing, it would be suitable to clarify certain points: As said before, the dorsal-ventral dissociations described, respectively, for syntactic-semantic operations [16, 17] as a general rule agreed with the anatomical proposal of Hickok and Poeppel [19]. However, this last model tried to integrate different theoretical views, types of tasks, methodological approaches, as well as different samples, including patients and healthy participants. Moreover, Hickok and Poeppel [19] predominantly reviewed the auditory and motor representations of speech, explicitly, the processes of speech perception and speech production whereas Catani and Bambini [16] and Hagoort and Indefrey [17] predominantly reviewed verbal comprehension in healthy participants. Speech production was rather avoided in these last two models. [22]

Regarding the present work, 'verbal perception and verbal production' will be seen as equivalent to 'verbal comprehension and verbal expression'. At once, the conceptual distinction between the 'comprehension-expression' organization and the 'semantics- syntax' one will be (partly) justified.

The 'comprehension-expression' organization and the 'semantics- syntax' one involve two different systems of classification, which are not mutually excluding. If correctly validated, both are plausible systems of verbal organization and interpretation. Comprehension involves both semantics and syntax, and the same applies to expression. Simultaneously, and if semantics and syntax are in fact psychologically dissociable processes, semantics would involve both comprehension and expression, and the same would apply to syntax (e.g., if the evaluation begins with syntax, then syntactic comprehension and syntactic expression will have to be evaluated). Within this line of reasoning, if comprehension and expression neurobiologically overlap it would be expectable that semantics and syntax also overlap.

---

[22] To be more specific: Hagoort and Indefrey [17] conducted a meta-analysis of neuroimaging studies which dealt with sentence comprehension in healthy participants; Catani and Bambini [16] also reviewed neuroimaging studies but mainly pointing at the recent advances in tractography, Catani and Bambini [16], on the other hand, also incorporated some PPA observations.

Alternatively, there is a frequent confusion between comprehension and semantics on the one hand, and between expression and syntax on the other hand, which will not be discussed here. Both systems of organization are interlaced but different. When people are verbally expressing or comprehending something, they are using the resources of semantics and syntax.[23] But when semantics and syntax are established as the initial and broader categories of analysis, then verbal comprehension and expression will function as their sub-categories or components.

There are also some pragmatic differences between both systems of classification: Unlike the dissociation between comprehension and expression, the dissociation between semantics and syntax is not easy to observe even using complex linguistic evaluations. Maybe this is so because the semantics-syntax organization was more conceptually conceived and used in academic and linguistic settings where, still today, there is debate about the differences between semantics and syntax. The concepts of autonomy, assessment, hierarchy, interdiscipline, models of evaluation and interpretation, among other topics, are still discussed in relation to semantics and syntax. Additionally, some new neurobiological models on the matter tend to exclude comprehension and expression from analysis even though the psychological dissociation between those two functions is naturally conceived and observed by any person. Parents, teachers, caregivers, nurses, and so on may frequently say: 'he/she understands everything but he/she can speak almost nothing' when referring, e.g., to two-year-old children or to patients with nonfluent aphasia. It is not necessary to be a neuroscientist to understand the concepts of verbal comprehension and expression. (Obviously, it is also simpler for neuroscientists to understand, explore and operationalize those concepts than the concepts of semantics and syntax). Accordingly, it is common knowledge that the behavior of verbal comprehension appears earlier in the ontogeny than verbal expression. As well, it can be observed in clinical settings that comprehension is usually recovered before expression after brain injury, and that comprehension is a strong condition for social adaptation and for recovering expression: if comprehension is not considerably (and quickly) recovered, the prognosis for the patient is poor.

Considering some pragmatic differences between both systems of classification in the field of aphasia, it is logically and empirically plausible to

---

[23] Vice versa cannot be that naturally said because semantics and syntax cannot be directly observed as behaviors.

verify the following statement:[24] 'without comprehension, it cannot be a coherent expression', which is true (see below). It is also logically and empirically plausible to verify that 'without a coherent expression, it cannot be comprehension', which is false; nonfluent aphasia is an example.[25] Unfortunately, similar statements are difficult or impossible to verify in the 'semantics-syntax' system, and this difficulty goes beyond the field of aphasia. For example, the affirmation: 'without semantics, it cannot be a coherent syntax' is dependent on the position in which both concepts are pondered. For example, for authors who consider that syntax is underpinned on the underlying semantic intention or perception, the statement is true. For those who consider that syntax is a formal reasoning, the first part of the statement (the antecedent) is irrelevant and, so, the statement itself is irrelevant. For those authors who consider that the antecedent and the consequence are relevant, the statement will only be logically and empirically verifiable if the sentential syntax is considered along with its semantic content. Under such circumstances, authors specifically verify what happens with or without semantics. The other way around ('without a coherent syntax, it cannot be semantics') is also difficult to analyze.[26] For example, and even for authors who, avoiding radical views, specifically verify what happens with or without a coherent syntax [17], it is difficult to say if the supposedly syntactic associations are in fact syntactic or semantic associations (see above the 'semantic consequences' of some syntactically coherent (and conventional) sentential examples [17]).[27] In any case, the semantics-syntax system is logically and empirically more complex and devious to analyze than the comprehensive-expressive system.

In spite of this, and considering the new neurolinguistic models on the matter [16, 17] it seems that, while the dissociation between comprehension

---

[24] Of course, comprehension, expression, semantics, and syntax are not dichotomous variables. The examples are specified with didactic purposes to show the complexity of comparisons. Besides, all those concepts are not equivalent.

[25] It could be said that, in the particular case of nonfluent aphasia, the function of comprehension acts rather independently of the function of expression.

[26] If: 1) semantics is considered synonymous with the whole sentential meaning, and: 2) a coherent syntax with such concept of semantics is considered synonymous with 'a sentence', then the sentential semantic unit (or gestalt) cannot be reduced to its elementary units. For radical views, there will be radical outcomes. E.g., for authors who consider that a coherent syntax (as a formal reasoning) is responsible for the meaning of any sentence, the statement is true.

[27] See also the definition of 'a sentence' given in the initial comments of this article, in particular for non conventional syntactic structures.

and expression is not reflected in anatomical sites, the dissociation between semantics and syntax is, anatomically, clearly observed.

Beyond such widespread (and amazingly consistent) neurobiological findings, the psychological interpretations about the semantics-syntax system remain ambiguous.

Hagoort and Indefrey [17], for example, affirm:

> 'Given that speaking and listening have different processing requirements, the same areas may not be recruited to the same degree in these two cases ... This difference between speaking and listening, however, does not detract from the finding that when needed, the same areas subserve unification operations in language production and language comprehension. Even less clear is the degree of separation between networks for syntactic and semantic unification.' pp 350 [28]

However, Hagoort and Indefrey [17] finally conclude:

> '...there is strong evidence for shared circuitry for core aspects of sentence-level language production and comprehension' thus confirming once more that the key psychological aspects to understand the neurobiological basis for language are semantics and syntax, although it is not psychologically quite clear what they are.' pp 359.

Regarding this issue, some unanswered questions will remain: If semantics and syntax cannot be psychologically and unquestionably dissociated (or the dissociation depends on theoretical/ abstract linguistic taxonomies, rather than on objective behaviors); why are semantics and syntax neurobiologically dissociated? Why are the neurobiological findings taken as evidence of the psychological dissociation between semantics and syntax thus discarding their interaction? Neurobiologically speaking: Why comprehension and expression overlap but semantics and syntax do not overlap if all these functions are not mutually excluding? Is it possible that researchers are measuring linear versus nonlinear neurolinguistic processes, or sequentially-perceived versus simultaneously- perceived semantic units? The underlying epistemological viewpoint will determine the way of validation of all these functions, and their interactions, in future studies.

[28] See above (in a footnote) the meaning of 'unification.'

Some Questions about Aphasia Analyzed within the New Epistemological Framework

Trying to ignore all the disquisitions expressed above regarding the characteristics of semantics and syntax, and trying to assume that: a) semantics and syntax do not differ in quality (explicitly, that they are comparable linguistic processes), b) the parts and the whole are equally important for both processes, and c) all the factors which eventually differentiate both processes can be manipulated by controlling experimental commands and conditions, two consequences for the aphasia topic can be proposed:

1) Patients with nonfluent/agrammatic aphasia (who supposedly have morphosyntactic impairments) cannot form words or bigger verbal constructions correctly. Maybe these patients can sometimes utter isolated words or even isolated sentences correctly but the rule is that they cannot properly form words, sentences and so on. That is so because they cannot link the components of those units. [29] Beyond the fact that agrammatism in itself implies that some words are missing, if it is also assumed that these patients really have morphosyntactic impairments, then they should have trouble with naming. However, in the PPA guidelines, for example, impaired naming is not described as a symptom for this type of aphasia [3]; patients with nonfluent/ agrammatic aphasia only have 'inconsistent speech sound errors' for otherwise semantically correct units. That is so even though the observational boundary between sound errors and phonological errors is diffuse: Both types of error may produce phonetic /phonemic paraphasias of any size (including small scale problems such as difficulties with a single sound or letter per word).[30] On the other hand, it would be incorrect to reason that patients with

[29] Just as a comment: The impaired comprehension of syntactically complex sentences is considered by some authors a symptom of nonfluent aphasia (see, e.g., [3]). In our experience, it may be a common disturbance of brain injured patients in general; it is not pathognomonic of patients with nonfluent aphasia and, so, it is not a valid construct for this aphasia. Reciprocally, patients with any type of aphasia usually have many cognitive domains impaired [9, 29].

[30] Some deficits described in the PPA guidelines [3] are difficult to verify; for example: 'effortful, halting speech with inconsistent speech sound errors…' which belongs to the agrammatic variant, versus 'speech (phonologic) errors in spontaneous speech …' which belongs to the logopenic variant. These deficits are not usually shown by means of empirical definitions in PPA studies, thus leaving to the discretion of each observer the final interpretation.

nonfluent/agrammatic aphasia show a correct speech just for semantic units at the single-word level because the lack of fluency can go from subtle impairments to mutism, thus covering a wide range of expressive semantic impairments. This range would go from simple word-distorting phonemes, morphemes (of any type) passing through single-words, to finally reach sentences, paragraphs, and so on. Or from the opposite perspective, if it is assumed that these patients do not have semantic impairments, then any semantic unit should be preserved, which is false. Sentences and words are incomplete, disorganized, and distorted because the whole expression is imprecise and nonfluent. Additionally, if the syntactic analysis is defined as a superior mechanism which organizes the inferior level of semantics [16, 17], when the superior mechanism is affected, the inferior one will become disorganized. I.e., if syntax is affected, semantics will be affected.

Independently of the above said and trying to understand this position, it could be thought the following: Cognitive functions which are less crystallized, less frequently used, more complex, or later acquired, tend to be the most vulnerable to brain injury. If that is so, and considering that syntactic ability is a late acquisition; is it probable that only the most formal details of verbal language are affected in patients with nonfluent/agrammatic thus producing a less sophisticated speech? If this temporal gradient really exists for syntactic functions; is there a possibility that nonfluent aphasia could be a less severe aphasia -rather than a different type of aphasia- in relation to the fluent one [34]?[31] Or from the opposite perspective, if it is assumed that semantics (which include nonverbal and multimodal signifier and signified sub-systems) is a more extended, crystallized, and resistant linguistic function in the brain; is it possible that all such neurolinguistic system inhibit the (pure semantic) naming errors in nonfluent aphasia? If this neurofunctional gradient really exists for semantic functions; is there a possibility that nonfluent aphasia could be a less severe aphasia -rather than a different type of aphasia- in relation to the fluent one?

Regarding just syntactic expression, it is difficult to understand the affirmation of Catani and Bambini [31] that there is one single restricted area

[31] Accordingly, is there a possibility that nonfluent aphasia could be the first to appear and/or the more frequent aphasia?

in the brain which triggers verbal fluency.[32] According to that finding, the frontal aslant tract would activate morphosyntactic concatenations not only independently of the rest of the cognitive functions, but also independently of grammatical or repetition deficits. By assuming that such excitatory (pure frontal) site exists [16, 31]; is it possible that its inhibitory counterpart is verbal comprehension [34]? If the ability of action monitoring (see Bonini et al. [36] quoted by Catani and Bambini, [16]) is conceptually added to the function of pure verbal fluency of the frontal aslant tract, then it could be deduced an inhibitory counterpart for pure verbal fluency.[33] Obviously, that would be so on the assumption that action monitoring [36] also encompasses verbal language monitoring. Without going so far, and by only considering the verbal language system, if it is assumed that comprehension involves an extended brain network in the left hemisphere, comprehension can be such inhibitory counterpart.

2) Patients with fluent aphasia (who supposedly have impairments in the most basic semantic units), cannot retrieve words and cannot understand the meaning of those words correctly. Maybe these patients can speak a lot, or link many verbal units; maybe the quantity of language production is adequate or even exacerbated, but the rule is that the quality of utterances is incorrect. As a result, these patients can neither utter words nor form bigger verbal constructions correctly: Paraphasias of any type, confusion between previous and subsequent words within a sentence, confusion between previous and subsequent phonemes/ sounds within a word; 'word salad', jargon, intrusions, perseverations, as well as circumlocution, anomia, and word-finding difficulties can be observed in patients with fluent aphasia. As they cannot retrieve and understand single words, more so they cannot retrieve and understand relationships among multiple words. Curiously, some authors believe that these patients have preserved syntax [3]. However, if the most basic semantic units are ambiguous, disordered or absent; how can they be uttered without affecting syntax? Patients with fluent/ semantic aphasia cannot have a 'fluent

[32] Peterson and Hagoort [35] affirm: 'For language, as for other cognitive functions, the function-to-structure mapping as one-area-one-function (as currently conceptualized) is likely to be incorrect. Brain regions typically participate dynamically as nodes in more than one functional network…'

[33] It is worth remembering that the frontal aslant tract does not belong to the level of syntactic analysis in the model of Catani & Bambini [16],

> language' because they cannot name and/or comprehend, among other impairments. They show substitutions, omissions, inversions, distortions and so on for phonemes, graphemes, words (of any type), sentences and bigger verbal constructions. Yet, and considering PPA [3] it is stated that, in the semantic variant, syntax is spared. Wilson, et al. [37] affirm that 'syntactic deficits can be defined as limitations in syntactic processing, which may be manifest in production, in comprehension, or most typically, in both production and comprehension.' Subsequently, those authors affirm (with 'robust body of evidence') that in most patients with semantic variant PPA, syntactic processing is strikingly spared. However, and considering more experimental paradigms [5, 17], even if patients are recruited [5], syntax can only be evaluated if semantics is spared.

Returning to the relationship between fluency and aphasia [31] previously analyzed in nonfluent aphasia, it is reasonable to conceive that, in fluent aphasia, the function of fluency is triggered in view of the lack of comprehension. Nevertheless, as the articulation or linking mechanisms (in the same way as the word retrieval mechanisms) cannot be monitored and amended, an appropriate sequence in the units of the language cannot be expected either. Interestingly, if there is a brain site which triggers verbal fluency independently of its quality (i.e., 'how much' a person speaks independently of 'how well' [38, 39]), that could explain why patients with fluent aphasia speak neither accurately in the semantics nor in the syntax.[34]

Unlike the expressed in the preceding paragraph, and trying to understand the affirmation of Wilson, et al. [37] regarding syntactic preservation in the PPA semantic variant, it could be thought the following: Although the ability to retrieve words and the ability to link words are mechanisms with an important automated component, maybe it is effortless to bring awareness the syntactic linear rules than the semantic nonlinear ones, e.g., it could be effortless to remember that an article comes before a noun than to unravel the intricate (and more automated) semantic relationships among word families. Even assuming that the syntactic rule might be perfectly retrieved by these means, the interaction with the retrieval of the rest of words cannot leave

[34] Analyzing the PPA guidelines [3] it seems that patients with nonfluent aphasia only have problems with the quantity of expression, and patients with fluent aphasia only have problems with the quality of expression. Quantity and quality were used in the item: Evaluation of Spontaneous Speech in the Brief Aphasia Evaluation [38, 39] but the deficit was analyzed, in this case, as a combination of both attributes.

aside. Under such circumstances, patients might be able to use syntactic structures but all types of erroneous words will be placed inside those structures. For example, articles will be searched from the semantic family of article words which, for having fewer options (and less complexity) than the family of nouns, will yield fewer errors than nouns but, finally, the organization of sentences will be affected by the use of multiplicity of quasi articles followed by quasi nouns and so on.

In summary, and even using the new way of thinking, it is expectable that nonfluent aphasia shows semantic problems and fluent aphasia shows syntactic problems. It is also possible that there is just a degree difference between both aphasias.

Aphasia and Some of Its Methodological Controversies under the Present Work Perspective

Taking into consideration the comprehension-expression system and studying samples of patients and healthy participants, Vigliecca and Baez [29] carried out an integrative (empirical) study addressed to obtain better definitions for verbal functions and sub-functions including: a) their organization under a hierarchical model, b) a lesion-based approach, and c) the analysis of a homogenously verbal and short aphasia test. Using confirmatory factor analysis and the Brief Aphasia Evaluation (BAE), a valid explanatory model for the neuropsychological characterization of aphasia" was proposed.

The model encompassed [29]:

a) An all inclusive verbal organizer from which two successive organizers emerged.

The two successive organizers were:

b) A more general classification which essentially included verbal comprehension and expression, in addition to a "complementary" verbal factor which included praxia, attention, and memory.

c) A more specific classification which included the individual (and correlated) constructs of auditory comprehension, repetition, naming, speech, reading, writing, and the "complementary" functions.[35]

By following this approach (where the aphasia patterns are exhaustively analyzed) all the patients fall inside the classification system; consequently, the gradual improvement of the aphasia theory is guaranteed. On the contrary, when only certain types (and number) of aphasias are considered as valid, without empirically demonstrating why other combinations of symptoms are not, the double dissociation which otherwise would be explicit becomes impossible to verify. The present probabilistic approach allows verifying this type of dissociation because any combination of symptoms is detected (and shown) and the theoretical interpretation is not left to chance. Additionally, as any pattern of the latent language impairments can be recognized, neurorehabilitation professionals are able to work with the particular characteristics of the patient, without being forced to follow a predetermined diagnosis typology. The model proposed in that work may represent a valid tool in the attempt to find new classifications or constructs for aphasia disorders (and their biological causes) beyond some widespread definitions and typologies [29].

New models concerning aphasia definitions, classifications, and their relationship with brain networks are necessary in particular because, so far, serious methodological inaccuracies can be verified in the available models.

Despite significant improvements observed in the psychological methods during the last years, the psychological outcomes are still puzzling. In the Publication Manual of the American Psychological Association [40], the methodological need of describing in detail the variable conceptual and operational definitions is stated. However this is not fully respected, particularly in clinical settings.

If the conceptual and the operational definitions are confused, the theory gets into an endless loop in view of the lack of distinction between conceptual agreement and real proofs [4, 26]. As concepts are still used during the phase of empirical validation, the hyper production of pseudoscientific articles becomes facilitated. Additionally, the use of typical cases seriously restricts progress [41].[36]

---

[35] It is worth noting that, except for the "complementary" functions, all the underlying verbal constructs follow the behavioral order of appearance in the ontogeny.

[36] This trend to use typologies can be illustrated with an analogous example in which three socioeconomic levels have to be empirically defined by using 15 supposed indicators [41]:

By using the method of selecting patients according to quantitative suggestions such as: 'at least one of these criteria', 'criteria X to Y must be absent', 'at least 2 of 3 criteria', etc., patients are actually grouped according to the number of present indicators (from zero to all the indicators). Although this method may produce hundreds or thousands of groups, experts only consider less than a handful of groups, which are in fact just 'the typical cases'. As the empirical/ operational definition is not exhaustive, the classification of 'the real cases' is impossible to be accomplished. Finally, the typical-case classification is exclusively made by expert-based evaluation.

'Under a correct empirical definition, all the cases should be feasible of classification but if real persons are confounded with ideals, many cases will be left out. That is why conceptual definitions should not be used for empirical demonstrations' [26].

When certain psychological qualities are intentionally selected to construct a 'typical' pattern so that such pattern agrees with what is expected by a theory, the pattern is constructed *a priori* and the research is biased. I.e., when only the diagnosis categories which confirm the syndromic hypothesis are included, the work is not scientific because there is no way of verifying the actual syndromic pattern in either the excluded cases or the compulsorily included ones.

In the case of aphasia, if only certain combinations of indicators are taken as the key ones for classifying patients in just, let's say, three aphasia categories (of the thousands of possibilities), then, those three categories will be at once the conceptual and the operational definitions. That is so because the patients' real responses are forced to go to those three conceptual categories. Since the categories of the dependent variable are constrained to be, as much as possible, the three initially conceived, methodological circularity is produced.[37]

This methodological difficulty can be seen in a paragraph taken from Mesulam, et al. [2]. The paragraph shows that 20% of the patients were (empirically) chosen to be included in the (conceptually) predetermined categories, namely, agrammatic (PPA-G), semantic (PPA-S), and logopenic (PPA-L) variants, in order to improve subtyping during demonstration. I.e.,

If inexperienced evaluators are involved, they will tend to define just three 'cases': the typical multimillionaire, the typical representative of the middle class, and the undeniable poor. Thus, almost 0% of all the possible cases would be classified.

[37] Even the empirical definitions of the Western Aphasia Battery have not been exhaustively constructed since the cut-off points do not consider all the possible combinations among symptoms [42].

these authors went back to the concepts during the result section of the study, more specifically, during 'the empirical validation of the classification guidelines', even if the quantitative criteria (the tests, the cut-off points and the empirical definition) had already been selected. Mesulam, et al. [2] wrote the following theoretical interpretations in the Results (instead of writing them in the Discussion):

> 'The classification guidelines of Table 1 lead to some ambiguity in differentiating PPA-G from PPA-L. For example, a patient with agrammatism, impaired repetition, impaired single-word retrieval and phonemic paraphasias would fulfil the criteria for both variants as long as motor speech, single word comprehension and object knowledge are spared. Thus, Patients 5, 8, 15, 17 and 20 fulfilled criteria for PPA-G as well as PPA-L. We chose to include_the former two in the PPA-G group because of the prominent agrammatism and the remaining three in the PPA-L group because we interpreted the exclusionary criterion number 4 for PPA-L in Table 1 ('absence of "frank" agrammatism') specifically to designate 'prominent' abnormalities of grammaticality, such as those that should lead to overt morphosyntax errors in speech' [2] pp. 1544.

Apparently, by applying a combination between the empirical definition and the clinical/ conceptual one, subtyping was improved. In this work, the authors wanted to test whether the recently published classification guidelines for subtyping PPA into agrammatic, semantic and logopenic subtypes [3] could be applied to patients with mild impairment. Regarding this outcome and the overlapping criteria for agrammatic and logopenic subtypes of primary progressive aphasia, Mesulam et al. [2] affirm: 'Quantitative criteria were least effective in the distinction of the agrammatic from the logopenic variant and left considerable latitude to clinical judgment.'

This is an example in which the division between the theory, the methods, and the results is not clear. Moreover, if patients' recruitment is based on this combination between the empirical definition and the conceptual one (instead of being based on an independent empirical definition) most of the cases of the dependent variable will be the theoretically expected ones.

To stop contaminating the results of the instruments (the real patient's data) from previous conceptual definitions [4], the deductive inference from the concepts to the symptoms (the empirical indexes) should come first and, at the end of the research, separately, the inductive inference (the interpretations) from the symptoms to the conceptual syndromes. Otherwise, the initial syndromic typology may become unalterable and the exhaustivity of the potential aphasia patterns (the real syndromes) may be lost.

The most convenient way to improve the aphasia theory is to incorporate all the mixed cases in the classification, which is equivalent to say that 'all' the patients are included. Since most of the patients have mixed (not typical) clinical manifestations [1, 41, 43], all the response possibilities have to be collected. If a psychological technique has the appropriate psychometric properties, a simple sum of scores is sufficient to cover all the response possibilities and get a correct empirical definition. Since such definition has to be made with the instruments of each laboratory, there cannot be a universal empirical/ operational definition. Additionally, the use of different empirical approaches serves to ensure that the scientific progress does not stay fixed under a dominant position. 'Unfortunately, most of the clinical definitions of typical syndromes have passed down from generation to generation based on tradition and agreement rather than on demonstration.' [29]. It is expected that this trend changes with the improvement of psychological methods.

Although, methodologically speaking, there is not much difference between the variants proposed in the PPA guidelines [3] and those proposed in the classical aphasia syndromes [44, 45], the PPA classification uses more indicators (from 8 to13 approximately, instead of 6) thus increasing the number of possibilities of combining symptoms and forming syndromes (from 256 to 8,192 possible syndromic groups, instead of 64 [46]). Since impairments in semantic and syntactic functions are included in the PPA guidelines, experts had to incorporate more indicators to assess those symptoms. Additionally, and even if pure language impairments are extremely frequent in the scope, experts are compelled to combine symptoms to form more complex syndromes to respect the theoretical guidelines, e.g., a patient with semantic aphasia has to show troubles with naming 'and' comprehension. In the work of Mesulam et al. [2], 12% of the patients were not classifiable by the PPA guidelines. The authors stated: 'All three stood out because of pronounced abnormalities in object naming. They came close to fulfilling the criteria for PPA-S except that word comprehension was preserved.' Obviously, this would not happen under a suitable operational definition. The 20% quoted above, and the 12% quoted here would be included.

In the psychological typology proposed by the so-called classical approach, various language functions are simultaneously evaluated in order to detect typical aphasia syndromes or pure language impairments. Four basic language functions (repetition, comprehension, expression, and naming) and two complementary ones (reading and writing) are usually studied as the elementary aphasia constructs or symptoms. However, at least eight aphasia syndromes (Broca, Wernicke, conduction, anomic, transcortical sensorial, transcortical motor, transcortical mixed, subcortical) and at least three pure language impairments (alexia, agraphia, verbal deafness) are deduced from the elementary constructs. While the elementary constructs are at most six, the diagnoses are at least eleven. Yet, the diagnoses keep increasing because they have not been exhaustively defined and many aphasia patterns fall outside the classification system [47].

A similar increase of syndromes can also be observed for PPA in just four years: Three [3], four [2], or even six [31] variants (the semantic, logopenic, nonfluent, and/or agrammatic as well as the mixed and severe ones) have been described. Considering the 12% excluded above [2] maybe anomic aphasia could be computed as the seventh variant.

Recently, Mesulam and Weintraub [48] wrote a commentary (with the name: 'Is it time to revisit the classification guidelines for primary progressive aphasia?') in which they said:

> 'Hair-splitting details of syndromic classification can hardly be expected to attract much attention. As in all areas of science, however, sound nosology and uniform nomenclature are important for progress in neurology. This is particularly true for the neurodegenerative syndromes, including primary progressive aphasia (PPA), where heterogeneity of phenotype and cellular pathology has defied attempts to coherent clinicopathologic correlations.' pp 1108.

The commentary was about an article of Wicklund et al. [49] where it was studied how well the consensus criteria could classify subjects with primary progressive aphasia (PPA) by following a quantitative approach. Thirty one percent of participants with a neurodegenerative speech and language disorder could not be classified, and twenty percent showed apraxia of speech without aphasia. The authors conclude: Application of consensus PPA criteria yields the three syndromic variants but leaves a large proportion unclassified. Therefore, the current consensus criteria need to be modified in order to improve sensitivity.

At the same time Mesulam et al. [50] observed that:

> 'Individual features of the aphasia, such as agrammatism and comprehension impairment, were as informative of underlying pathology as more laborious subtype diagnoses. At the single patient level, no clinical pattern was pathognomonic of a specific neuropathology type, highlighting

the critical role of biomarkers for diagnosing the underlying disease. During clinical subtyping, some patients were unclassifiable by the 2011 guidelines whereas others simultaneously fit two subtypes. Revisions of criteria for logopenic primary progressive aphasia are proposed to address these challenges' pp 1176.

As shown in these quotations, psychological assessments are not relevant by themselves. Apparently, they can only be estimated as relevant if they help to find biological markers.

The syndromes of the PPA guidelines [3] were proposed to divide the clinical manifestations of PPA based on specific speech and language features characteristic of each subtype. However, if all of those theoretical syndromes have never been psychologically validated, they cannot be used as the gold standard for validating other measures addressed to assess, precisely, those syndromes (see, for example, Agosta et al. [33], described above).

In addition, aphasia patterns have to be discovered independently of their biological basis in order to avoid circularity. Nevertheless, this is impossible to do if brain imaging, neurobiological/ neurofunctional patterns, and/ or other biological indices are put together with the psychological patterns in the consensus diagnosis guidelines.

THE 'OLD-FASHIONED' VIEW OF PSYCHOMETRY

A psychological disorder and its biological causes cannot be established by convention.

The impetus to reach agreement with psychological events has led to the shocking situation in which a consensus-criterion article published in 1984, for example [51], has been quoted almost 22,000 times by April of 2015 as synonymous with the procedure for demonstrating diagnosis. Considering the guidelines of 2011 for primary progressive aphasia, that number was almost 800 in just four years [3].[38] As such psychological criteria were established by authority, its 'validity' does not require demonstration. Subsequently, clinicians and researchers are authorized to diagnose and treat patients without any other requirement than quoting those criteria. Within a certain clinical

[38] For researchers who have been formed with an experimental approach that situation is at least irregular. Methodological quality and reasoning have lost value in favor of the quantity of information as well as the reproduction (rather than the renovation) of contents and approaches.

topic, there will basically be a single guiding criterion (excluding the almost identical ones), until the experts meet again. At the same time, journal reviewers usually demand that such criterion is quoted in the articles. In such a way, all the material and human resources are put at the service of the guiding consensus proposal, being the resources put at the service of getting *post-hoc* empirical validation the most noticeable.

Validity in psychology is usually confused with agreement, and agreement is usually confused with empirical consistency. By this mean, the intersubjective consensus of experts becomes a 'theory' and the subsequent studies will tend to confirm it, with minor details. As previously explained, all this occurs because the pattern of the patient's psychological data is conceptually (not empirically) built. Finally, the supposed consistency is magnified by dissemination.

A theory should be defined as 'scientific' by its method, not by its content, not by its data-collection techniques and, much less, by the name of its authors or its widespread application. Present consensus definitions are essentially based on literature reviews as well as the number of publication of the authors involved. Unlike consensus, a proposal based on logical and mathematical principles is independent of prestige.

Since prestigious subjectivity is a more powerful subjectivity, the initial (well-intentioned) attempt to avoid psychological subjectivity turned out to be counterproductive: An incorrect epistemological structure is worldwide encouraged to be the same from the beginning to the end of the research so that the choices lean toward staying in the same conceptual system. Considering that without change there is no improvement, scientific knowledge is hindered.

In the 'consensus' articles it is usually written: a) the psychological diagnosis was made by some expert X according to the consensus definition Y,[39] b) the technique Z (which generally represents the originality of the research) was applied to the diagnosed groups, and c) the results are ...

Since no demonstration is needed for the first step, neither expertise nor the consensus definition is empirically verified [4]. Regarding psychological diagnosis, the question that arises is the following: If it is true that all the corresponding psychological instruments have been applied for diagnosis; why their results are not (completely) shown?

[39] If the theory is not valid, and the supposed expert is functional to the theory, then the expert can turn out to be inexpert for other theories. He/ she may not be able to see the variable categories and clusters of the other theories and, so, there may be (unintentional) bias due to such singular expertise.

Fortunately, the manifestations of psychological disorders are increasingly demanded to be more objectively proven. Such methodological demand is probably bringing about a little more frequent emergence of proposals aimed to renovate the consensus criteria. These proposals are refreshing since it is expected that literature reviews and, particularly, diagnosis guidelines change all the time according to the renewal of empirical findings. However, this change is very slow in view of the redundant framework on which the prevailing viewpoint rests. At present, and considering the new methodological demands, maybe the question expressed above has to be reformulated as follows: If the psychological results have to be shown; why the predetermined patterns of responses appear practically indistinguishable at the beginning and at the end of the research?

When reasoning is wrong it can be anticipated that the results will be wrong, but when most of the studies tend to confirm the consensus theory, something serious occurs, something that exceeds (or makes useless) scientific methodology and logics.[40]

Nowadays, there are a lot of coincident reviews with 'undisputable' inferences where brain images are highlighted as a sort of (psychological) validation procedure in itself. It is quite the opposite view of the classical aphasia approach when the brain images were absent. Between both extremes of such an imaginary pendulum, the validity of psychological tasks and experimental designs remain obscure. In both extremes, psychological interpretations and preconceptions are dominant. Besides, scientific reviews seem to be captive of previous renowned findings. Although pioneering works and their authors are remarkable, that is not a reason for repeating them indefinitely. Moreover, if attention is not paid, this may be a way of getting stuck.

Even if dissent and the questions which cannot be answered by the present theory are the keys for generating scientific progress, they are usually avoided. On the contrary, there is a sort of constant search for consistency and widespread validation. Article reviews must look for similarities and differences but, for some reason, reviewers tend to seek similarities as much as possible.

[40] It can be useful to remember that expert-consensus overvaluation was one of the causes of the scientific impasse in the middle age. At the present time, and considering the problems generated by the globalization, Science must be more than ever independent of the Establishment. However, proposals and articles of renowned scientists and journals have now become synonymous with better and forced-to-be-quoted ones. They represent 'the' dissertations of reference.

Twenty five years ago Summers and Lederman [52] wrote something that is applicable to the present time and topic: 'Literature reviews... emphasize positive results, down-playing the null findings and extensive methodological inadequacies in the published...studies.'

Additionally, the link between psychosocial and biological sciences has created new challenges. For example, the direct transference from medicine to psychology of the methodological structure to construct nosologies has lead to considering psychological symptoms as if they were physical. But psychological symptoms need to be first translated to 'physical signs' (to put the expression in medical words) in order to be objectively assessed and then, secondarily, interpreted. Such translation is the operational definition. The association observed between a measure obtained with a biological technique and a measure obtained with a psychological technique is not equivalent to the translation of psychological symptoms or syndromes to observational 'signs'.

The ability to link psychological aspects with more organic (and supposedly more objective) substrates has produced a sort of euphoria that tend to obscure the fact that psychological aspects remain today as difficult to assess as throughout history. The validation of one psychological symptom is complicated, but the validation of several syndromes is much more complicated. Yet, the proposal of psychological syndromes is rife these days. The biologistic trend is predisposed to believe that psychological events are quite 'freely negotiable', until a biological marker appears.

If the interaction between medical and psychological nosologies do not involve logical reasoning for deciphering the genesis and organizational structure of their concepts, including the basic distinction between the independent and dependent variables [4], the interdisciplinary efforts might enter into a speculative vortex similar to the observed in very ancient times or in the always present psychological pseudoscience.

Operationalization is part of the standard procedure to develop psychological studies and instruments. It is a useful step to deduce objective evaluations from concept/ consensus definitions; thus, it is a necessary step within each research which involves psychological assessment. Unlike the concept/ consensus definitions, which rely on authority, the validity of the psychological operational definitions does require empirical demonstration. However, with the advent of the clinical definitions by consensus (paradoxically presented as 'operationalizations') the specific study of the psychological assessment has lost status and high impact journals are not interested in psychometrics. On the contrary if a revolutionary neurobiological technique interacts with a psychological outcome, the research will be interesting, no matter the details of the psychological assessments, if they are shown at all.[41] Nevertheless, the neurobiological techniques also require validation and, curiously, such validation comes from psychology. Since the concurrent validity involves a two-way implication, the psychological validation is a necessary condition for demonstrating the neurobiological one.

A valid conceptual classification for aphasia symptoms and syndromes (or verbal functions and their organization), according to biological evidence, is necessary not only for discovering the dissociations and interactions among neuropsychological functions, but also for studying the consistency among different approaches, samples and instruments. This theoretical model should go beyond the novelty of the circumstantial instrument used for data collection, require deep methodological considerations and, if so, it will result in better research, therapeutic or preventive proposals. Neuropsychology has two parts. When article reviews are done, the psychological validity of tests and experimental designs has to be analyzed along with the neurobiological outcomes. If the consistency among neurobiological outcomes is based on doubtful psychological outcomes, the theoretical inferences will be doubtful.[42] To be more specific, if the validity of the psychological outcomes is doubtful, any language neurobiological model will be doubtful.

A correct approach in the field of aphasia demands that the psychological symptoms and clusters of symptoms are defined in relative terms so that the interaction with lesions and clusters of lesions can be established by demonstration. Although there are some new attempts of modeling the relationship between brain and language, they mainly accentuate bibliographic and neurobiological consistency. I.e., psychological manifestations and interpretations can apparently remain open (or secondary) in view of the neurobiological evidences. Maybe for this reason the neurobiological evidences are so consistent while the psychological ones are not.

---

[41] The confusion between the validation of the psychological assessments, on the one hand, and the validation of the study itself, on the other hand, also produces confusion among all the steps and procedures involved in the research. For example, if it is stated in the Methods, that the independent and dependent variables to be shown in the Results are highly correlated, the only step left for the rest of the research will be to describe the results of the already known correlation. It is very common these days that psychological assessments and their properties are *ad hoc* shown, wherever they become more convenient. Therefore, they can be at once the cause and the consequence.

[42] Currently, most of the authors seem to share the approach which goes from psychology to neurobiology. Beyond the fact that, for aphasia (and by definition), the opposite direction should prevail, it would be interesting to see more frequently the exploration of the verbal-language functions as dependent variables: from neurobiology to psychology.

Psychometry helps to discover the validity of the instruments as well as the dissociations and interactions among psychological functions. In clinical settings, for example, if the consensus guidelines state that other cognitive disturbances have to be dissociated from aphasia, such dissociations have to be shown in the research. Beyond the guidelines, if a certain test is proposed to assess, e.g., grammatical- processing, and the test involves reading, the dissociation which demonstrates that grammatical- processing is independent of reading has to be shown.

The contribution of psychometrics to the neurosciences in general and to the aphasia theory improvement in particular has to be reconsidered. The feedback that exists between theory and instrument is best understood under this perspective. Although the instruments are based on the theory to prove their validity, they simultaneously serve to improve the validity of the theory. To avoid that this virtuous circle becomes a vicious one, all the steps of the scientific method has to be respected and dissociated from each other. As seen above, this objective is far from being achieved.

Considering aphasia diagnosis, only when the patterns have been consistently validated through different laboratories and approaches, they can be proposed as a theory. Otherwise it may be more useful to continue just with the symptoms.

REFERENCES

[1] Sinanović O, Mrkonjić Z, Zukić S, Vidović M, Imamović K. Post-stroke language disorders. *Acta Clin. Croat.* 2011; 50(1):79-94.

[2] Mesulam MM, Wieneke C, Thompson C, Rogalski E, Weintraub S. Quantitative classification of primary progressive aphasia at early and mild impairment stages. *Brain.* 2012; 135(Pt5):1537-53.

[3] Gorno-Tempini ML, Hillis AE, Weintraub S, Kertesz A, Mendez M, Cappa SF, Ogar JM, Rohrer JD, Black S, Boeve BF, Manes F, Dronkers NF, Vandenberghe R, Rascovsky K, Patterson K, Miller BL, Knopman DS, Hodges JR, Mesulam MM, Grossman M.Classification of primary progressive aphasia and its variants. *Neurology.* 2011; 76 (11):1006-14.

[4] Vigliecca, NS. Dementia and mental disorders: Methodological considerations. In Goldfarb PM, (Ed.), Psychological tests and testing research trends. New York: Nova Science Publishers; 2007; pp 177-188.

[5] Tyler LK, Marslen-Wilson WD, Randall B, Wright P, Devereux BJ, Zhuang J, Papoutsi M, Stamatakis EA. Left inferior frontal cortex and

syntax: function, structure and behaviour in patients with left hemisphere damage. *Brain.* 2011; 134(Pt 2):415-31.

[6] Rayner K, Duffy SA. Lexical complexity and fixation times in reading: effects of word frequency, verb complexity, and lexical ambiguity. *Mem. Cognit.* 1986;14(3):191-201.

[7] Tyler LK, Marslen-Wilson WD. The on-line effects of semantic context on syntactic processing. *J. Verb Learn Verb. Beh.* 1977; 16: 683–92.

[8] Marslen-Wilson W, Tyler LK. The temporal structure of spoken language understanding. *Cognition.* 1980; 8(1):1-71.

[9] Viglieсca NS, Peñalva MC, Molina SC, Voos JA, Viglieсca MR. Is the Folstein's Mini-Mental test an aphasia test? *Appl. Neuropsychol. Adult.* 2012; 19(3):221-8.

[10] Burgess, A.; Sherman, B. (eds.): Metasemantics: New Essays on the Foundations of Meaning. Oxford: Oxford University Press; 2014.

[11] Corominas-Murtra B, Fortuny J, Solé RV. Towards a mathematical theory of meaningful communication. *Sci. Rep.* 2014; 4:4587.

[12] Horn, L.; Ward, G. (eds.): Handbook of Pragmatics, Oxford: Blackwell; 2004.

[13] Jackendoff, R.: Foundations of language: brain, meaning, grammar, evolution. Oxford: Oxford University Press; 2002.

[14] Kiss, T.; Artemis, A. (eds.): Syntax Theory and Analysis. An International Handbook. Handbooks of Linguistics and Communication Science. 42 (1-3). Berlin: Mouton de Gruyter; 2015.

[15] Murphy, B.: A Study of Notions of Participation and Discourse in Argument Structure Realisation. Dublin: Trinity College Dublin; 2007.

[16] Catani M, Bambini V. A model for Social Communication and Language Evolution and Development (SCALED). *Curr. Opin. Neurobiol.* 2014; 28:165-71.

[17] Hagoort P, Indefrey P. The neurobiology of language beyond single words. *Annu. Rev. Neurosci.* 2014; 37:347-62.

[18] Hickok G, Poeppel D. Neural basis of speech perception. *Handb Clin. Neurol.* 2015; 129:149-60.

[19] Hickok G, Poeppel D. Dorsal and ventral streams: a framework for understanding aspects of the functional anatomy of language. *Cognition.* 2004; 92(1-2):67-99.

[20] Milner, AD. & Goodale, MA.: The visual brain in action. Oxford: Oxford University Press; 1995.

[21] Saj, A; Vuilleumier, P.: Agnosias, apraxias, and callosal disconnection syndromes. In: Caplan, LR. & van Gijn, J. (eds.) Stroke Syndromes, 3rd

edition. Cambridge, UK: Cambridge University Press; 2012; pp. 267-286.

[22] Wright P, Randall B, Clarke A, Tyler LK. The perirhinal cortex and conceptual processing: Effects of feature-based statistics following damage to the anterior temporal lobes. *Neuropsychologia.* 2015; pii: S0028-3932(15)00048-2.

[23] Kelleher, J; van Genabith, J.: *A* computational model *of the* referential semantics *of* projective prepositions. *In:* Saint-Dizier P. (ed.) Syntax and Semantics of Prepositions. Text, Speech and Language Technology, vol. 29. Netherlands: Springer; 2006; pp. 211–228.

[24] Newman AJ, Pancheva R, Ozawa K, Neville HJ, Ullman MT. An event-related fMRI study of syntactic and semantic violations. *J. Psycholinguist. Res.* 2001; 30(3):339-64.

[25] Col G, Aptekman J, Girault S, Poibeau T. Gestalt compositionality and instruction-based meaning construction. *Cogn. Process.* 2012; 13(2):151-70.

[26] Vigliecca, NS. Are Vascular, Alzheimer and Mixed Dementias Distinctive Entities? In: SR Jacobsen (Ed.), Vascular Dementia: Risk Factors, Diagnosis and Treatment,. New York: Nova Science Publishers; 2011; pp 177-188. See also the same title [online]. 2011 [cited 2015, June 19]. Available from: https://www.novapublishers.com/catalog/product_info.php?products_id=21998

[27] Burgoon, JK; Buller, DB; Woodall, WG. Nonverbal communication: The unspoken dialogue (2nd ed.). New York: McGraw-Hill; 1996.

[28] Guerrero, LK; Floyd, K. Nonverbal Communication in Close Relationships. New Jersey: Lawrence Erlbaum Associates, Inc.; 2005.

[29] Vigliecca NS & Báez S. Verbal Neuropsychological Functions in Aphasia: An Integrative Model. *J. Psycholinguist. Res.* 2015; 44 (6): 715-732.

[30] Brauer J, Anwander A, Perani D, Friederici AD. Dorsal and ventral pathways in language development. *Brain Lang.* 2013; 127(2):289-95.

[31] Catani M, Mesulam MM, Jakobsen E, Malik F, Martersteck A, Wieneke C, Thompson CK, Thiebaut de Schotten M, Dell'Acqua F, Weintraub S, Rogalski E. A novel frontal pathway underlies verbal fluency in primary progressive aphasia. *Brain.* 2013; 136 (Pt 8):2619-28.

[32] Malaia E, Newman S. Neural bases of syntax-semantics interface processing. *Cogn. Neurodyn.* 2015; 9(3):317-29.

[33] Agosta F, Ferraro PM, Canu E, Copetti M, Galantucci S, Magnani G, Marcone A,Valsasina P, Sodero A, Comi G, Falini A, Filippi M.

Differentiation between Subtypes of Primary Progressive Aphasia by Using Cortical Thickness and Diffusion-Tensor MR Imaging Measures. *Radiology. 2015*; 141869.

[34] Vigliecca NS, Báez S, Griffouliere ME.Broca's aphasia: a different type of aphasia or a less severe aphasia? [online]. 2012. [cited 2015, June 19] Available from: http://www.conicet.gov.ar/new_scp/detalle.php?keywords=&id=19856&congresos=yes&detalles=yes&congr_id=1534868

[35] Petersson KM, Hagoort P. The neurobiology of syntax: beyond string sets. *Philos Trans. R. Soc. Lond. B. Biol. Sci.* 2012; 367(1598):1971-83.

[36] Bonini F, Burle B, Liégeois-Chauvel C, Régis J, Chauvel P, Vidal F. Action monitoring and medial frontal cortex: leading role of supplementary motor area. *Science.* 2014; 343(6173):888-91.

[37] Wilson SM, Galantucci S, Tartaglia MC, Gorno-Tempini ML. The neural basis of syntactic deficits in primary progressive aphasia. *Brain Lang*. 2012; 122(3):190-8.

[38] Vigliecca, N. S. (2000). Brief aphasia evaluation (BAE) [Database record]. *PsycTESTS.* [cited 2015, June 19] Available from: http://psycnet.apa.org/?&fa=main.doiLanding&doi=10.1037/t16313-000

[39] Vigliecca, N. S. (2000). Evaluación Breve de la Afasia (EBA) [Database record]. *PsycTESTS*. [cited 2015, June 19] Available from: http://psycnet.apa.org/?&fa=main.doiLanding&doi=10.1037/t24812-000

[40] American Psychological Association (APA). Manuscript Structure and Content. In Publication Manual of the American Psychological Association (6th ed.) Washington, DC: APA.; 2009; pp. 29.

[41] Vigliecca NS; Báez S. The homeless millionaire, the illiterate with a lofty status and the ever-present influence of stereotypes and beliefs in the course of science [online]. 2014. [cited 2015, June 19] Available from: http://www.conicet.gov.ar/new_scp/detalle.php?keywords=&id=19856&congresos=yes&detalles=yes&congr_id=4253407

[42] Vigliecca NS, Peñalva MC, Molina SC, Voos JA. Brief Aphasia Evaluation (minimum verbal performance): Concurrent and Conceptual Validity Study in Patients with Unilateral Cerebral Lesions. *Brain Injury.* 2011; 25 (4), 394-400.

[43] Vigliecca NS, Peñalva MC, Molina SC, Castillo JA, Vigliecca MR. Aphasia: when the minority is the norm [online]. 2011. [cited 2015, June 19] Available from: http://www.conicet.gov.ar/new_scp/detalle.php?keywords=&id=19856&congresos=yes&detalles=yes&congr_id=1957238

[44] Goodglass, H; Kaplan, E. Evaluación de la afasia y de trastornos relacionados. Madrid: Panamericana; 1996.

[45] Shewan, CM., & Kertesz, A. Reliability and validity characteristics of the Western Aphasia Battery (WAB). *J. Speech Hear Disord*. 1980; 45 (3), 308–324.

[46] Viglìecca NS. Aphasia: What are we measuring? [online]. 2010. [cited 2015, June 19] Available from: http://www.conicet.gov.ar/new_scp/detalle.php?keywords=&id=19856&congresos=yes&detalles=yes&congr_id=1815517

[47] Viglìecca, NS. Aphasia: When just one neuropsychological condition generates more syndromes than symptoms [online]. 2010. [cited 2015, June 19] Available from: http://www.conicet.gov.ar/new_scp/detalle.php?keywords=&id=19856&congresos=yes&detalles=yes&congr_id=1815516

[48] Mesulam MM, Weintraub S. Is it time to revisit the classification guidelines for primary progressive aphasia? *Neurology*. 2014; 82(13):1108-9.

[49] Wicklund MR, Duffy JR, Strand EA, Machulda MM, Whitwell JL, Josephs KA. Quantitative application of the primary progressive aphasia consensus criteria. *Neurology*. 2014;82(13):1119-26.

[50] Mesulam MM, Weintraub S, Rogalski EJ, Wieneke C, Geula C, Bigio EH. Asymmetry and heterogeneity of Alzheimer's and frontotemporal pathology in primary progressive aphasia. *Brain*. 2014; 137 (Pt 4):1176-92.

[51] McKhann G, Drachman D, Folstein M, Katzman R, Price D, Stadlan EM. Clinical diagnosis of Alzheimer's disease: report of the NINCDS-ADRDA Work Group under the auspices of Department of Health and Human Services Task Force on Alzheimer's Disease. *Neurology*. 1984; 34(7):939-44.

[52] Summers DC, Lederman SJ. Perceptual asymmetries in the somatosensory system: a dichhaptic experiment and critical review of the literature from 1929 to 1986. *Cortex*. 1990; 26(2):201-26.

In: Aphasia
Editor: Christina T. Rogers
ISBN: 978-1-63483-993-8

Chapter 2

ACQUIRED CHILDHOOD APHASIA: A MOSTLY UNKNOWN PHENOMENON

Dr. Melanie Kubandt[*]
University of Osnabrueck, Department of Education,
Section Early Childhood Education, Osnabrueck, Germany

ABSTRACT

Acquired Childhood Aphasia (ACA) is a medical phenomenon which is still mostly unknown and often disregarded. One reason for this disregard is the rarity of aphasia in children often being emphasized, and the prognosis being assumed to be more favorable for children and adolescents than for adults. Another common reason for the disregard is the lack of understanding the clinical picture of aphasia in children. The provided chapter offers a broad overview of possible definitions, symptoms, prognosis and outcomes of Acquired Childhood Aphasia and the impact on quality of life for the affected children and adolescents and their families. It goes on to show that the prognosis is not as favorable as often proclaimed, and impacts the affected children and their families in numerous ways. Finally, this chapter points out possibilities of therapeutic intervention and provides examples of measures of support for the families.

[*] melanie.kubandt@uni-osnabrueck.de

Introduction

There are numerous reports and research papers on aphasia, or at least on the variety affecting adults. Reports and papers on Acquired Childhood Aphasia (ACA), however, are still being marginalized. Globally speaking, there's the occasional research, notably stemming from Anglophone countries; compared to research papers on adult aphasia, however, are few and far between. This marginalization of ACA encompasses not only the fields of aphasiological research and education, but also the subsections of diagnostics and therapy. However, the last twenty years have shown discernible efforts to intensify research in this particular area of aphasiology. Various authors have repeatedly drawn attention to the lack of knowledge and research concerning the etiology and concepts of ACA diagnosis and therapy in recent decades. Presently, there's a discernible and increasing focus on ACAs acting as a spotlight on the phenomenon.

Aphasias in Children and Adolescents - Definitions

A pervasive, yet not undisputed criterion for defining aphasia is the completion of language acquisition. However, aphasias are most definitely not limited to adults possessing a complete vocabulary. Damage to the brain, predominantly by way of traumatic brain injury (TBI), can lead to sudden-onset acquired aphasia in children and adolescents (cf. Leischner 1987, Rother 2005, Spencer 2006): "Like adults, children can exhibit language disorders from injury to the central nervous system after a period of normal development. Childhood-acquired language disorder, or childhood-acquired aphasia, refers to language impairment evident after a period of normal language acquisition that is precipitated by, or associated with, an identified form of brain insult." (Dennis 2010, p. 418). Dennis and Barnes (1990) state that head injury is the most common form of acquired brain damage in children and adolescents. Spencer (2006) regards TBI as the leading cause of acquired aphasias in childhood and adolescence, with a prevalence of 80% (cf. Hécaen 1983, Leischner 1987, Paquier/Van Dongen 1993). According to Siegmüller and Heide (2006), children suffer traumatic brain injuries primarily through vehicular accidents, through falling down whilst playing or doing sports or as a consequence of physical violence: "The neurobiology of childhood traumatic brain injury (TBI) includes immediate impact injury (contusions, diffuse axonal damage), secondary intracranial events (hematomas, brain swelling, infections, subarachnoid hemorrhages, hydrocephalus), and extracranial factors (hypoxia, hypotension). TBI results in focal brain damage (vascular injury involving contusions and hemorrhage, especially in the frontal and temporal lobes) and diffuse brain damage (to axons in the white matter), as well as in secondary damage such as raised intracranial pressure, hypoxia, and ischemia" (Dennis 2010, p. 418).

While strokes constitute the most common cause of aphasias in adult patients (in 80% of cases), resulting in unilateral focal lesions, children tend to present with diffuse, most commonly bilateral injuries affecting several cerebral areas to a variable extent. Granted, strokes can also occur in children, but this is among the rarely observed causes of ACA (cf. Spencer 2006).

ACAs show a marked difference in appearance, progression and pathogenetic conditions when compared to aphasias in adults (cf. Poeck/Hacke 2006, p. 102). Among the other possible causes of ACAs are brain tumors, degenerative diseases of the central nervous system, encephalitis and epilepsy (cf. Becker et al. 1986; Fabbro 2004).

Dennis and Barnes (1990) point out: "Recent studies of language in head-injured children and adolescents have concerned three issues: The rate of language recovery; the relationship to language deficits of factors like age, etiology, lesion size, and lesion site; and the form and range of the clinical language disturbances." (ibid. p. 429). If the cerebral language disorder's causes are pre- or perinatal, the affected children won't be able to complete a regular language development. These cases are not referred to as ACA. Some authors roughly differentiate childhood language disorders as either 'disorders of speech development' or 'ACAs' (cf. Leischner 1987, p. 268; Rother 2005, p. 90). According to Leischner (1987), these can be further delineated: A disorder of speech development commences at a time when linguistic development has either not yet begun or has not yet been completed. ACA, in contrast, can be defined as the loss of an already acquired faculty of speech, analogous to adult aphasia (cf. Leischner 1987, p. 268). Therefore, only postnatal injuries can by definition be regarded as the cause of ACA (cf. Van Hout 1992; Rother 2005). To what extent aphasias can occur prior to the conclusion of linguistic development, however, is left ambiguous in Leischner's delineation. In contrast, there are authors who choose to apply the term of ACA to impaired children who have not yet completed their language development (cf. Friederici 1984). This approach has asserted itself in recent years. In this regard, however, Rother (2005) as well as Leischner (1987) emphasize the necessity of aphasia being defined as the degeneration or loss of pre-existent faculties of speech (cf. Rother 2005, p. 91). Van Hout (1992) includes this facet in her by now generally accepted definition of ACA: "(1) An acquired lesion must have occurred after a lesion-free period, a free interval, and thus differs from the lack of language of congenital dysphasias in which the insult is pre- or perinatal; (2) Some normal language must already have been present, the accepted age-dependent boundary usually being 2 years of age, the time of the advent of the first sentences." (ibid. p. 140). In practice, children are therefore regularly being diagnosed as aphasic even before the completion of language development. The linchpin of this definition is the proficiency in language production. Fabbro (2004) concurs with Van Hout's definition and adds: "Acquired childhood aphasia refers to language deficits following brain lesions after the age of acquisition of the first sentences, generally after the age of 2." (ibid. p. 1). This illustrates among other things a fundamental distinction in regards to disorders of speech development, seeing as childhood aphasias are the result of a distinct incident.

Acquired Childhood Aphasia – Not That Common?

Oftentimes, ACA is and has been labelled as a rare disorder. There exist no precise figures with regard to its prevalence and incidence. Guttmann (1942) however casts doubts on the relative rarity of the clinical picture, based on studies conducted more than 70 years ago: "[I]t is surprising that the rarity of aphasia in children is so often emphasized, and I think this can be accounted for only by lack of understanding of the clinical picture of aphasia in children" (ibid. p. 208). Compared to adult-centric aphasiology, Guttmann defines the problem of diagnosis thusly: "Aphasia in the adult is mostly diagnosed or sought for when the patient complains of difficulty in his speech – which children do not do – or if he uses wrong names for objects; in other words, apart from cases of complete motor aphasia, the early diagnosis of aphasia is commonly based on subjective or objective word-amnesia. The clinical appearance in children is different, and the signs of aphasia in a sick, apathetic, shy and often morose child are easily overlooked unless specially sought." (ibid.).

Satz and Lewis (1993) share these doubts and point towards studies indicating a higher number of children exhibiting aphasic symptoms than commonly being estimated in professional circles. Grimm (2003) states as well that about 2% of children exhibiting language impairments should actually be regarded as ACA sufferers. Hécaen (1983) even goes as far as to posit: "Aphasia is more frequent, at least among the youngest children, than in adults." (ibid. p. 581).

In summary, concerning the evolution of aphasiology with regards to child-specific language impairments, the following can be ascertained: Starting with the earliest accounts of ACAs and up to the late 1970s, aphasiological research was concerned only with atypic manifestations of the clinical picture (cf. Guttmann 1942; Basser 1962; Alajouanine/Lhermitte 1965), or at least emphasized it in contrast to the heterogeneity of adult aphasia. Thus, ACA was primarily defined as nonfluent aphasia commonly occurring in confluence with lesions of the right hemisphere (cf. Paquier/Van Dongen 1998). On top of that, the notion of a swift and complete convalescence in ACA sufferers was purported for a long time (cf. Guttmann 1942; Basser 1962; Alajouanine/Lhermitte 1965; Lenneberg 1967; Hécaen 1976). Aphasia in adults and ACA were long distinguished by three main criteria: "(1) The children`s symptoms were said to be uniform and predominantly nonfluent, whatever the lesion localization; (2) Prognosis was assumed to be more favourable for children than for adults; (3) The frequency of right-hemisphere lesions was thought to be higher in children than in adults." (Van Hout 1992, p. 139).

This perception of ACA has nonetheless shifted gradually since the late 1970s. Analogous to the research on aphasias in adults, there exist group studies (cf. Clarus 1874; Guttmann 1942; Alajouanine/Lhermitte 1965; etc.) as well as case studies (cf. Holland 1970; Lehecková 2004; Martins 2004 etc.). One singularly important medical innovation was the emergence of medical imaging, precipitating new insights regarding ACA. Employing computer-assisted tomography, Loonen and van Dongen (1990) determined the confinement of anomalies to the left hemisphere in the entire sample of aphasic children examined by them – a notion that had long been contested. Similarly, the techniques of PET, MRI and SPECT were more frequently employed over time (cf. Paquier/van Dongen 1998, Dennis 2010). Contrary to the established belief in the homogeneity of nonfluent ACA's clinical picture, regardless of lesion location (cf. Guttmann 1942), these studies illustrate the correlation of lesions in various left-hemisphere regions with varying syndromes of aphasia (Paquier/van Dongen 1998).

SYMPTOMATOLOGY IN ACA

Dennis (2010) points out that children show a range of language disorders after acquired brain injuries and that language breakdown may occur at the level of pragmatics, semantics, syntax, morphology, phonology, or speech production. Thus, the clinical presentation of ACA affects all areas of language competence, just as it does with adult aphasia. In this context, it's important to note that both forms of aphasia involve loss of language faculty and language comprehension based on cerebral organic causes, usually concomitant with retention of functionality in organs of speech, auditory perception and intelligence (cf. Kubandt 2009).

The traditional concept of ACA was primarily informed by the symptom of "nonfluency" as with Broca's aphasia in adults (cf. Bernhardt 1885). This concept assigned five principal characteristic traits to ACA: Mutism, a period of hypospontaneity of speech, dysarthria, agrammatism and so-called "negative signs" (Van Hout 1992, p. 146). Negative signs, in this case, are conceived as the absence of symptoms usually occurring in adult fluent aphasia, like jargon, logorrhea, paraphasia, neologism etc.

Traditional concepts regard *mutism* as one of the main symptoms of ACA. Branco-Lefévre (1950) and Alajouanine and Lhermitte (1965) assumed a period of mutism ensuing immediately after the onset of an aphasic disorder. Likewise, Hécaen (1976) determined that such a period of mutism lasts far longer in ACA patients than it does in adults. He further stated a correlation between the type and location of cerebral injuries and the emergence of mutism. In this regard, von Cramon (1981) distinguishes between two different types of mutism: "true mutism" denotes the inability of expressing any sounds at all, while "word mutism" describes the inability of expressing oneself verbally resp. communicating (cf. ibid. p. 801ff). The term "aphasic mutism" is commonly used instead of "word mutism," though it's often difficult to distinguish from the so-called period of *"hypospontaneity of speech"* (cf. van Hout 1992, p. 146; Satz/Lewis 1993, p. 650f.), meaning a decrease in spontaneous speech, which often follows the period of mutism. This period usually lasts longer than mutism (cf. Satz/Lewis 1993). The symptomatology also encompasses a deficiency in initiating conversations. This phenomenon is rarely found in adult aphasic patients and is also considered as characteristic for ACA (cf. van Hout 1992). It is furthermore prevalent in young children. Van Hout and Seron (1983) regard the dysfunction of a speech "initiator" in connection with subcortical structures as the root cause of this symptom (ibid. p. 193). Spencer (2006) describes the decrease in spontaneous speech as a limitation and simplification of verbal behavior, as a depletion of vocabulary, as a reduced rate of speech and as a diminished mean length of utterances (MLU).

Deficiencies in the area of syntax have been an issue since ACA was first reported (cf. Bernhardt 1885) – however, there has not yet been enough research conducted in this field. Alajouanine and Lhermitte (1965) proceed on the assumption that syntax in aphasic children is characterized by simplification rather than deficiency, as is the case with aphasia in adults suffering from *agrammatism.* It is for this reason they state that "true agrammatism never occurs in children" (ibid. p. 658). Boehringer et al. (1979) too declared there to be no similarities to adult agrammatism. In contrast, Dennis (1980) assumes that agrammatism can very well occur in children and impair expressive as well as receptive capabilities. One problem in diagnosing agrammatism relates to the fact that due to mutism resp. reduction of spontaneous speech, the MLU in aphasic children often turns out to be rather sparse. This in turn exacerbates the effort of drawing conclusions with regards to syntactic abilities. On a lexical level, ACA sufferers display conspicuous problems in naming things (cf. Satz/Lewis 1993). In his 1983 studies, Hécaen observed lasting "naming disorders" in 44% of ACA cases with left-hemisphere lesions (cf. ibid. p. 58ff). Cases like this are commonly referred to as *anomies* (cf. Van Hout 1992; Satz/Lewis 1993). Moreover, the following is held to be true with regards to ACA-induced lexical disorders: "Lexical problems have been described as true anomia, reduced with the help of phonemic cues, or as a *loss* or poverty of vocabulary, more similar to a reduction of use or an impoverishment of the memory stock." (Van Hout 1991, p. 118).

Concerning the existence of paraphasias, professional opinions differ. As well as disputing the existence of childhood agrammatism, Alajouanine and Lhermitte (1965) also deny the occurrence of paraphasias with regards to ACA, or at least emphasize its scarcity (cf. ibid. p. 658). Hécaen (1976) aligns himself with this notion. More recent studies however produce arguments for the existence of paraphasias (cf. Van Hout et al. 1985; Visch-Brink/Van de Sandt-Koenderman 1984; Van Dongen/Visch-Brink 1988). They offer a possible explanation for the counterargument of scarcity by pointing out that paraphasias in conjunction with ACA mostly occur over only a short period of time and thus are more likely to be overlooked (cf. Satz/Lewis 1993). According to Aram (1991), paraphasias are much more likely to emerge in acute phases, but might also persist over a longer period of time. Spencer (2006) as well assumes that semantic and phonemic paraphasias present themselves primarily in the first few months following a child's impairment. Dennis and Barnes (1990) have shown that children with TBI have deficits in comprehension of mental state verbs as well. As mentioned earlier, traditional doctrine regarding ACA presupposed the existence of so-called *"negative signs"* until the end of the 1970s. The notion of these "negative signs," encompassing for example mutism, dysarthria, telegram style and a reduced length of sentences, led to a characterization of ACA as predominantly "non-fluent" (cf. Fabbro 2004). Guttmann (1942), Alajouanine and Lhermitte (1965) as well as Hécaen (1976) even assumed a complete absence of fluent aphasias in children. This traditional concept, however, has been amended by several studies conducted in recent years. In this context, Aram (1991) drew attention to the dearth of crucial information with regards to the language of aphasic children: "Very little systematic investigation of phonology or articulation has been pursued among children with acquired aphasia; the data are not available to generalize as to conditions that may relate to the presence or absence of phonological and/or articulatory problems." (ibid. p. 437).

Hécaen (1976) refers to impairments of *written language* as frequently occurring in ACA sufferers. According to Alajouanine and Lhermitte (1965), disorders of written language acquisition are generally encountered in the context of ACA and more prevalent than linguistic disorders. All three authors point out that ACA in conjunction with written language is far more likely to affect writing disorders than impairments in reading proficiency (cf. Alajouanine/Lhermitte 1965; Hécaen 1976). Spencer (2006) describes it as the worst possible partial prognosis, taking into consideration that reading and writing are the last acquired modalities of language acquisition. In this context however, Aram (1991) criticizes the lack of detailed reports and studies regarding written language proficiency in afflicted children. Even if it is less impaired than written language proficiency, reading proficiency is often significantly more dysfunctional than spoken language. On the other hand, Dennis (1980) was able to show by means of a study that while reading proficiency was much more impaired than language proficiency during the acute phase of affliction, those circumstances underwent a reversal over the course of three months. One has to bear in mind though that, according to Rother (2005), in the context of writing and reading dysfunctions are particularly noticeable if these skills were already acquired premorbidly (cf. ibid. p. 52). Some studies however show that children who have acquired aphasias at a pre-school age are faced with significant issues, meaning they either won't be able to learn how to read and write or merely on a very limited level (cf. Gloning/Hift 1979). In general, a correlation between the severity of written language impairment and the age of the afflicted children is hypothesized (cf. Rupp 2006). Thus, Hécaen (1976) observed deficiencies of written language in 90% of under-10-year-olds vs. only 45% of over-10-year-olds. Since younger children are still in the process of learning written language, they often display more severe difficulties. Aram (1991) too emphasizes how skills that have yet to be acquired are more susceptible to dysfunctions than those premorbidly existent. These cases are further aggravated by the difficulties in performing a differential diagnosis between aphasia and dyslexia, especially if the aphasia hasn't been recognized as such and the corresponding symptoms only appear years after the acquired cerebral impairment. All told, what can be established is that recent studies indicate a variety of different reading and writing dysfunctions as possible effects of ACA, comparable to those experienced by adult acquired aphasia sufferers (cf. Loew/Böhringer 2002, p. 23).

Utilizing new techniques and improving upon existing neurolinguistic testing procedures, it has now become possible to examine highly diverse aspects of language more accurately. Procedures such as these made it feasible to establish *"positive symptoms,"* like *logorrhea, paraphasias, perseverations* and *neologisms*, alongside the previously mentioned negative symptoms (cf. Fabbro 2004; Lehecková 2004; Paquier et al. 2004): "Recent case studies show a great variety of aphasic symptomatologies including auditory comprehension disorders, paraphasias, neologisms, logorrhea, jargon, impaired repetition abilities, and a host of linguistic deficits in reading and writing." (Paquier/van Dongen 1996, p. 428).

Thus, nowadays it has become basically assumed that all symptoms occurring in adults might also be found in children (cf. Van Hout/Evrard/Lyon 1985; Martins/Ferro 1991; Fabbro 2004; Lehecková 2004; Paquier et al. 2004; Rother 2005).

Compared to the vigorous efforts in classifying the various aphasic dysfunctions in adults however, there have been markedly fewer corresponding attempts with regards to ACA. Aside from classification in terms of etiology, lesion locus and manner of spontaneous language, ACA used to always be described and categorized via its symptoms (cf. among others Van Hout 1992): "The aphasic symptoms in children are not as differentiated with respect to location as in the adult." (Tartter 1998 p. 223; also cf. Goodglass 1980). One of the most current works on ACA, "Neurogenic Language Disorders in Children" (2004), edited by Franco Fabbro, nonetheless asserts that all adult-specific aphasic syndromes can also occur in children: "Moreover, these symptoms correlate with clinical aphasic profiles and lesion localizations similar to those of adults. Indeed, at least in their acute phase and lesional phase aphasic syndromes in children have been found similar to most of the aphasic syndromes in adults." (Fabbro 2004, p. 2). Likewise, Van Hout (1992) and Van Dongen et al. (2001) refer to the "existence of an adult-like heterogeneity of childhood aphasic syndromes." (ibid. p. 345). In this regard however, Van Hout (1992, 1993) points out that although aphasic symptoms in children have been found to be similar to those of adults, children may show atypical symptoms. Among professionals, this is considered status quo as far as the symptoms of ACA are concerned.

SYMPTOMS ASSOCIATED WITH ACA

Aside from aphasia, several other attendant symptoms may occur, among them for example hemiplegia, epilepsies, dysphagia and disorders of concentration, attention and memory (cf. Franke 2004). Hécaen (1976) and Leischner (1987) for example observed a high number of hemipareses in aphasic children. According to Spencer (2006), damage to the frontal lobe as a common result of traumatic brain injury can lead to attention disorders and disorders of the working memory in aphasic children, as the frontal lobe is host to these neuropsychological functions. In the context of ACA, Miller et al. (1984) address other characteristic traits not directly attributable to the aphasia. They determined that ACA often goes hand in hand with comprehension issues and note, among other things, that afflicted children oftentimes appear deaf-like and also act accordingly. Guttmann (1942) and Agranowitz/McKeown (1975) have also drawn attention to this particular aspect of ACA. Rothenberger (1986) observes that cognitive, motoric and emotional issues are possible byproducts of aphasia. Sollee and Kindlon (1987) see a correlation between cerebral lesions and behavioral problems in children, thereby corroborating studies conducted by Herzberg and Herzberg (1977). Campbell and Heaton (1978) too refer to behavioral disorders. To them, this includes diminished attention, aggression, temporary outbursts and, in some cases, hyperactivity. Agranowitz and McKeown (1975) also describe these phenomena and state: "Behavior problems play an important part in the diagnosis of aphasic children." (ibid. p. 192). Dennis and Levin (2004) discuss the behavioral outcome after TBI too. Mantovani and Landau (1980) suspect that behavioral disorders in connection with ACA "may reflect a primary disinhibition at limbic or diencephalic levels." (ibid. p. 528). In contrast, Miller et al. (1984) would sooner ascribe the behavioral problems to the sudden loss of speech and look towards psychological reasons as root causes. The studies of Campbell and Heaton (1978) also speak for the validity of the latter explanation. Their thesis is based on the observation that behavioral disorders tend to disappear once the afflicted children are presented with alternative systems of communication.

Furthermore, a syndrome often mentioned in context of ACA is the so called Landau-Kleffner-Syndrom. Bishop (1985) describes it as a "syndrome of acquired aphasia with convulsive disorder, in which language regresses after a period of normal development and seizure develop" (ibid. p. 705).

PROGRESSION, PROGNOSIS AND OUTCOME

Dennis and Barnes (1990) state that "the bases for language symptom patterns and recovery rates in children and adolescents with acquired lesions are poorly understood" (ibid. p. 429). Concerning recovery and linguistic capabilities of ACA sufferers, a marked variance in prognosis and progression is held to be true. The primary factors being recognized in connection with recovery are type of injury and age of the child at the lesion's onset (cf. Aram 1991). Progression of ACA has almost exclusively been characterized in relation to the question of prognosis. Despite numerous studies, the long-term development of ACA still remains ambiguous (cf. Miller et al. 1984). The traditional view of ACA proceeded from the assumption of an excellent prognosis, especially when compared to adult aphasia (cf. Clarus 1874; Bernhardt 1885; Freud 1897). This traditional notion endured over the course of the 20th century (cf. Guttmann 1942; Alajouanine/Lhermitte 1965; Lenneberg 1972; Hécaen 1976). The researchers arrived at this conclusion by way of the long-held assumption that aphasic symptoms in children were merely temporary and rarely persistent. In his study, Guttmann (1942) recounts astonishingly positive prognoses in some cases: "The recovery from aphasia of the purely motor type is surprisingly rapid, and most cases with a reversible lesion have recovered within four weeks." (ibid. p. 218).

More recent papers and studies on the topic contradict this hypothesis at least to some extent. For example, Satz and Bullard-Bates (1981) analyzed data on ACA that had been published up to 1978 and pointed out that 25 to 50% of cases were still suffering from aphasia a year after onset of the disorder. Loonen and Van Dongen (1990) observed comparable cases: "Most of the children had not recovered completely 1 year after onset." (ibid. p. 1324). Jordan and Murdoch (1994) examined a number of adults who had suffered severe head injuries during childhood and reached a similar conclusion: "Results indicated that all areas of language competence assessed (syntax, semantics, and pragmatics) appeared to be compromised by the childhood closed-head injury." (ibid. p. 506). Two years later, Jordan and Ashton (1996) published a similar study with a subject group comprised of children and arrived at the same results.

One possible explanation for these recent insights and notions may well be that earlier studies had either neglected to account for variables that could possibly affect the prognosis or had merely considered them in a fleeting manner. Van Hout (1991) criticizes the long-held belief of age being the main criterion for a good prognosis. She counts etiology, age at the time of onset, lesion scale and types of aphasia among the variables far more important for arriving at a prognosis. The differing etiologies of ACA render it nigh impossible to reach a universally valid assessment. The factor of differing etiologies being mostly disregarded might be explained by the long-held notion of childhood aphasias as relatively homogeneous phenomena. Van Dongen and Loonen (1977) were among the first to ascribe vital importance to etiology with regards to prognosis. Among other things, they reached the conclusion that ACAs stemming from cerebral traumata will often recover completely (cf. ibid. p. 135f). Moreover, they argued in favor of the prognosis of traumatically induced aphasias being much better than of those stemming from inflammatory processes. Niedergall and Remschmidt (1981) share this opinion. Dennis and Barnes (1990) state that "recovery of speech and language in instances of childhood head trauma is overall better than recovery from some other acquired conditions of childhood" (ibid. p. 429). Martins and Ferro (1991) however arrive at this conclusion: "[The] children with stroke had a very good recovery compared to those with traumata and especially the infectious cases." (ibid. p. 179). Dennis and Barnes (1990) conclude that "not all clinical language functions return after head injury. And even after clinical recovery of language, the question remains how effectively the individual can use language for social and interpersonal communication, a question that concerns not clinical language functions (naming, repetition, fluency, and the like), but discourse." (ibid. p. 429). A different case study of Martins (2004) based on fifty ACA patients indicates that in 11 cases, the patients were still suffering from chronic aphasia two years later. She thus concludes that it's not factors like age or gender that are of relevancy to the recovery process, but rather factors related to the scale and location of the lesion. One difference between ACA and aphasia in adults is the time of improvement, according to Martins: "Curves of aphasia recovery in adults (again, mostly stroke patients) have shown that the greatest improvement is seen in the first 3 months (especially in the first three weeks)... There may be some recovery during the first year..., but afterwards there are no significant changes, and functional decline has occasionally been reported... Although children who recovered did so during the first year, in our group of chronic aphasics improvement of different language abilities was found not only after the first year, but also 5 or more years after lesion onset, causing changes in the aphasic profile and taxonomic diagnosis." (ibid. p. 245). According to Martins, another fundamental difference with regards to adult aphasics' recovery lies in the fact that with children, language performances were far more likely to improve even in the chronic period: "Regarding recovery, there are two main differences between these findings and findings related to adult aphasics. First, unlike adults, the overall recovery was better in children and, secondly, children improved in the chronic period." (ibid. p. 245). Martins argues in favor of a better prognosis for ACA versus adult aphasia in general, yet criticizes the lack of knowledge regarding cases of chronic aphasia. Leheckovά (2004) arrives at a similar conclusion. By contrasting the recovery of a Czech child suffering from aphasia with that of an adult aphasia patient, she reasons thusly: "The child's aphasia is basically manifested in the same way as the adult's aphasia with one exception: while the adult patient two years post-onset reached a stage after which her language skills no longer improved, the child has continued to develop her linguistic abilities." (ibid. p. 227f).

All told, it is notable that ACA prognosis is not regarded as positively today as it once was, especially compared to adult aphasia. Factors like age and gender have taken a backseat to etiological factors.

Nevertheless, more recent studies demonstrate that even with existing resp. chronic aphasias, there is still the possibility of successful recoveries, especially in children. A number of authors attribute this fact to the brain's plasticity during childhood (cf. Becker et al. 1986; Loew/Böhringer 2002, Fabbro 2004). Even in this context however, the prognosis is not estimated as positively anymore as traditional notions once held (cf. Kubandt/Friede 2011).

In this context, one aspect that is left unconsidered by ACA research is the fact that in some cases, aphasic symptoms can still emerge long after the acute event and subsequently remain unrecognized. This could possibly be one cause of childhood and adolescence aphasias not being diagnosed (cf. Kubandt 2008a, 2009). Benz and Ritz (2003) thus call attention to the no longer applicable traditional adage positing that, due to the brain's plasticity, the long-term effects of TBI are significantly more favorable the younger a child is at the time of the accident. The authors argue that children actually tend to grow into their permanent deficit. Another aspect to consider with the so called phenomenon of 'growing into deficit' is the fact that afflicted children often experience retardation of further development. This results in a progressive ability gap when compared to their peers, one that subsists even in the face of continuous development. The issue has long been neglected and disregarded. In this context, the prognosis for ACA sufferers is negative insofar, as the afflicted need to both reacquire the abilities they have lost due to cerebral injuries as well as develop additional abilities to advance their overall progress. This in turn necessitates repeated examinations to supervise further progression following the accident or onset of disease (cf. Kubandt 2009).

All in all, and analogous to adult aphasias, ACA is not without consequences. Aside from the symptomatic impairments already mentioned, there are also *psycho-social consequences* to contend with. Unfortunately, this is another area that has so far been rather neglected by ACA research (cf. Kubandt 2008a). This leads Martins (2004) to emphasize the negative consequences of ACA in spite of its overall supposedly better prognosis compared to adult aphasia: "Although chronic aphasics tend to have mild forms of aphasia and their linguistic abilities may continue to improve in the chronic stage, persistent aphasia has a negative impact on their educational, social and professional life." (ibid. p. 247). The three mentioned aspects also play a vital part in the context of therapeutic interventions.

To summarize the phenomenon of ACA it can be referred to a definition by Brown and Hécaen (1976):

"1. Acquired childhood aphasia is characterized by mutism or agrammatism at an early age, and by anomia and nonfluent phonemic paraphasias somewhat later. 2. Articulatory disorders in acquired childhood aphasia appear in the context of a nonfluent or borderline fluent state. 3. The picture of fluent phonemic paraphasias in conversation (conduction aphasia) is rarely encountered. 4. Logorrhea and semantic or neologistic jargon do not occur in acquired childhood aphasia. 5. Disorders of comprehension are present in about one-third of the patients, but the adult-type correspondence between comprehension loss and logorrheic jargon is not found. 6. Recovery tends to be superior to recovery in adult aphasia. 7. At any early age, there is a relatively even chance that aphasia will occur with injury to either hemisphere." (ibid. p. 189).

PROSPECTS OF INTERVENTION REGARDING ACA

The area of clinical intervention is highly significant to people suffering from aphasia as well as their family members. There exists a wealth of research regarding diagnostics and therapy for adult aphasics. Just as in all other respects, aphasiology targeted towards children has, however, taken a clear backseat to adult-specific aphasiology. Instead, diagnostic and therapeutic tools designed with adults in mind are also employed with ACA, without ever having been empirically proven as beneficial (cf. Kubandt/Friede 2011). Within the fields of diagnostics and therapy, two main trends are predominant: Cognitive neurolinguistic on the one hand, offering a possible foundation for precisely structured and scientifically valid diagnostics and therapy; and, on the other hand, a pragmatic-communicative approach mainly allowing for diagnostic as well as therapeutic procedures in the context of communicative agency and daily routine (cf. Kubandt 2008a). Even today, literature on ACA very rarely references diagnostics and therapy. Seeking a similar range of diagnostic options and techniques as is typically on offer for adult aphasias proves to be a fruitless endeavor.

DIAGNOSTICS

Guttmann (1942) was among the first researchers to draw attention to the inherent difficulty in diagnosing ACA. Numerous cases remain undetected, which Guttmann regards as a reason for the general assumption of low prevalence. His definition of ACA posits the disease not as a rare occurrence, but rather as a seldom recognized clinical picture. Agranowitz and McKeown (1975) characterize these undiagnosed childhood aphasias as the single most serious issue for those persons affected by them.

Diagnostics in general aim to obtain as comprehensive an impression as possible of a child's linguistic abilities to use as a springboard for further therapeutic steps. This includes assessment of the pre-morbidly achieved level of speech (cf. Loew/Böhringer 2002, p. 29). On one hand, this assessment is necessary in children with acquired cerebral injuries in order to differentiate between a language impairment and ACA; on the other hand, it offers hints as to therapeutic strategies and their objectives. Furthermore, the pre-morbid level of speech (among other factors) can also offer indications concerning progression and prognosis. However, Becker, Bergmann and Kubiak (1986) emphasize that aphasic impairment may well be the most prominent symptom in children and adolescents, but hardly the only one. The cerebral injury negatively impacts the child's entire personality (ibid. p. 59). It is for this reason they call for examinations to assess a child's entire personality instead of merely cataloguing its linguistic abnormalities.

Practice has proved the usefulness of gathering essential information regarding the pre-morbid level of speech by way of initiating a dialogue with the parents and having them fill out questionnaires, as well as gaining access to school reports (cf. Kubandt 2008b). The checklist of diagnostics developed by Bulling, Geigenberger and Hofman (2002) can serve as one possible example of such a questionnaire. In it, questions regarding manners of speech and communication both pre- and post-onset are posed. In order to examine motor speech, screenings for apraxia of speech and dysarthria may be employed (cf. Loew/Böhringer 2002; Spencer 2006). Yet another aim of diagnostics is assessing the progression of the disease. Findings and information supplied by prior attending facilities and specialists, like rehab clinics, schools, physicians, neurologists and speech therapists for example, as well as statements from relatives, allow for more specific diagnostics. Information such as this is especially vital in diagnosing illusory recovered aphasias (cf. Chilosi et al. 2008). Beyond that, Loew and Böhringer (2002) regard the assessment of a child's current need for communication as an important diagnostic goal. Yet another aspect figuring into the issue of diagnostics is the assessment of other neuropsychological abilities - attentiveness and perceptiveness, for example. Becker, Bergmann and Kubiak (1986) point to the importance of not merely using the diagnosis to assess the impaired abilities and performances of the afflicted children, but above all those a child is still in possession of, since these serve as a gateway to rehabilitation (ibid. p. 59).

THERAPY IN APHASIC CHILDREN

With regards to therapy in aphasic children, there is much research still to be done, especially in direct comparison to the wealth of available therapeutic approaches and techniques for adult aphasia (cf. Kubandt 2009). Becker et al. (1986) cite rehabilitation of the linguistic abilities possessed by the child pre-insult as an integral task of therapy, as well as the acquisition of new linguistic skills (like written language skills, for example), since the latter usually poses considerable difficulties to the afflicted children (ibid. p. 63). They denote the exceptionality of ACA therapy vs. therapy for adult aphasia thusly: the conjunction of practices acting towards the recovery and acquisition of linguistic skills during an individually aggravated learning process (ibid). Eisenson and Ingram (1972) consider it of vital importance to diagnostically assess a child's pre-morbid level of linguistic development before the start of therapy, the former serving as a starting point for the latter. Therein lies a fundamental difference to rehabilitation in adults: While adult aphasia patients' therapy is geared mainly towards recovery of pre-existing skills, children are obligated to undergo further development in all respects, be it motorically, linguistically, socially or cognitively. Thus, it is not enough to merely relearn pre-morbidly existent skills. Consequently, the focal point of rehabilitation, in addition to the *reclamation* of pre-existent skills, is stimulating a child's capacity *to learn something new*. Both of these aspects are of central importance in ACA therapy and should be borne in mind.

Work with Parents

Relatives should receive information about the clinical picture of aphasia and act as significant support systems during therapy (cf. Becker et al. 1986; Spencer 2006): "Parents of the aphasic child are usually confused and baffled by the many problems confronting them." (Agranowitz/McKeown 1975, p. 196). This has the effect of further elevating the importance of working with parents in the context of therapy – not only to assist affected parents and siblings, but also the afflicted children themselves. Especially where aftereffects, like for example behavioral disorders, are concerned, educating parents resp. relatives becomes a substantial aspect of therapy: "The parents need to understand the basis of their child's behavior. Most of the symptoms are directly related to the brain injury and must be understood as part of the picture of the aphasic child." (ibid. p. 197) There should be parent counseling with regards to possibilities of the child's reintegration at school and the most advantageous course of education (cf. Kubandt 2008a, Kubandt 2009). Therefore, working with parents is regarded as a central aspect of the therapeutic process by all the authors. In this respect, Becker et al. (1986) consider both one-on-one conversations and parent group discussions as useful tools to be employed regularly in addition to a child's therapy. Agranowitz and McKeown (1975) recommend parent groups as a medium of reciprocal communication and support. Roberts (1966) likewise regards working with parents a fundamental pillar of therapy. Hahn et al. (2002) too conducted regular meetings with parents during the course of therapy in order to provide transparency and point out support options to them. They consider it just as relevant to create a setting for potential questions and issues on the parents' part and stressed the need to impart advice for dealing with a speech-impaired child (ibid. p. 50). The aims of meeting with parents outlined above are generally acknowledged as being sensible and should be considered for comprehensive use in therapy.

SCHOOL REINTEGRATION OF APHASIC CHILDREN AND ADOLESCENTS

A general question within the context of young patients' aphasia therapy is the one concerning their continued school career. The ICF's conception of target objectives in particular places the individual in its entirety in the centre of the rehabilitative process and regards scholastic and occupational rehabilitation as worthy goals in addition to medical rehabilitation. Becker et al. (1986) therefore recommend a therapeutic course of action within small groups of children, regarding it as preparation for an eventual rehabilitation of the aphasic child into the school system. Roberts (1966) and Haynes (1986) also recommend group-centric therapeutic measures.

The question of further scholastic development is of vital importance with regards to ACA, yet still remains sparsely researched (cf. Kubandt 2009), just like every other field of child-oriented aphasiology. Agranowitz and McKeown (1975) are among the few to have focused on this subject. They note that school should be adjusted towards the children's needs: "the aphasic child learns better in a situation with minimal stimulation." (ibid. p. 194). Another of the few publications on this topic originates from Girolami-Boulinier (1986) and addresses the scholastic development of children and adolescents in the Paris area. However, Girolami-Boulinier himself notes that this should by no means be considered a representative study. Its results are as follows: From the perspective of school education, a return to the past school system route is important (with or without delay). If an adolescent has not reacquired this former level after 1.5 to 2 years, it becomes necessary to detect possibilities of directing him towards an apprenticeship that actually corresponds with his interests, so his acquired skills won't deteriorate anew (ibid. p. 85). Admittedly, reintegration into regular school is often impossible since overly large grades and time pressure due to curricula do not allow for catering to the individual needs of impaired children. Hofmann Stocker (1991) determined by way of a study that of 23 adolescents suffering from aphasia, only half were able to resume their education. It is for this reason Birkenbeil (1995), in marked contrast to Girolami-Boulinier (1986), calls for specially tailored types of schools. In general, the question of school rehabilitation still remains insufficiently researched, with many problems left unsolved and many questions unanswered (cf. Kubandt 2008b, Kubandt 2009).

CONCLUSION

Regarding the field of aphasia research in the context of ACA, there's an evident future need for increased attention and efforts. A pivotal research gap concerns the field of diagnostics and therapeutic studies. The necessity of speech therapy is undisputed, yet there are no particular standardized testing procedures and therapy programs available, creating a rather significant need for further research. A particular problem in this regard is posed by issues of quality assurance, efficiency and effectiveness of diagnostics and therapy. At the present time, both diagnostics and therapy run the risk of arbitrariness. Means of interventions regarding ACA that are based on adult aphasiology pose the danger of outdated and heavily criticized approaches and materials being adopted for the purpose of children- and adolescent-oriented intervention, unreflecting and without regard for the criticisms voiced by researchers. At a time evidence-based rehabilitation is at the centre of debates, this seems problematic and academically untenable.

Regarding the demonstrated particularities of prognosticating ACA, the ultimate conclusion is to commence with the rehabilitation process of aphasic children and adolescents as soon as possible (i.e., directly following the acute clinical treatment) and to allow for a sufficient period of time. Furthermore, the process should be comprehensive, including medical measures as well as those with the purpose of scholastic, occupational and psychosocial rehabilitation.

REFERENCES

Agranowitz, A., & RiddleMcKeown, M. (1975). Aphasia Handbook for Adults and Children. Springfield: *C. C. Thomas.*

Alajouanine, Th., & Lhermitte, F. (1965). Acquired Aphasia in children. *Brain,* 88, 653-662.

Aram, D. M. (1991). Acquired Aphasia in Children. In: M.T. Sarno (Ed.), Acquired Aphasia (pp. 425 - 455). New York: *Academic Press.*

Basser, L. S. (1962). Hemiplegia of early onset and the faculty of speech with special reference to the effects of hemispherectomy. *Brain,* 85, 427-460.

Becker, R., Bergmann, B.-E., & Kubiak, I. (1986). Zur Rehabilitation aphasischer Kinder. In: R. Becker, & Elstner, W. (Eds.), Das aphasische Kind. Berlin: *nes.*

Benz, B., & Ritz, A. (2003). Besonderheiten bei der neurologischen Rehabilitation von Kindern und Jugendlichen: Seminarbericht "Neurologische Rehabilitation von Kindern und Jugendlichen," 07.-09.10.2003. Bremen: *Friedehorst.*

Benson, D. F. (1972). Language Disturbances of Childhood. Clinical Proceedings: *Children´s Hospital National Medical Center*, 28, 93-100.

Bernhardt, M. (1885). Ueber die spastische Cerebralparalyse im Kindesalter (Hemiplegia spastica infantilis), nebst einem Excurse über "Aphasie bei Kindern." *Archiv für pathologische Anatomie und Physiologie und für Klinische Medicin,* 102, 26-80.

Birkenbeil, C. (1995). Aphasie im Kindesalter. In: M. Grohnfeldt (Ed.), Sprachstörungen im sonderpädagogischen Bezugssystem. Handbuch der Sprachtherapie (pp. 405 - 419). Berlin: *nes.*

Bishop, D.V.M. (1985). Age of onset and outcome in acquired aphasia with convulsive disorder (Landau-Kleffner-Syndrome). *Dev Med Child Neurol* (6), 705-12.

Boehringer, J.C., Doms, M.C., & Fery, C. (1979). Erworbene Aphasie bei Kindern im Vorschulalter. In: G. Peuser (Ed.), Studien zur Sprachtherapie (pp. 222-235). München: *Wilhelm Fink Verlag.*

Branco-Lefévre, A. (1950). Contribuicao para o estudo da psicopatologia da afasia em criancas. *Arquivos de Neuro-Psiquiatria*, 8, 345-393.

Brown, J. W., & Hécaen, H. (1976). Lateralization and language representation. *Neurology,* 1976 Feb.26, 2, 183-189.

Bullard-Bates, C., & Satz, P. (1981). Acquired aphasia in children. In: M. T. Sarno (Ed.), Acquired Aphasia (pp. 399 - 426). New York: *Academic Press.*

Bulling, St., Geigenberger, A., & Hofmann, E. (2002). Checkliste für Diagnostik. In: M. Loew, & K. Böhringer (Eds.). Gailingen: *Hegau-Jugendwerk.*

Campbell, T. F., & Heaton, E.M. (1978). An expressive speech program for a child with acquired aphasia: a case study. *Canadian Journal of Human Communication, Summer*, 89-102.

Chilosi, A. M., Cipriani, P., Pecini, C., Brizzolara, D., Biagi, L., Montanaro, D., Tosetti, M., & Cioni, G. (2008). Acquired focal brain lesions in childhood: effects on development and reorganization of language. *Brain and Language,* 3 (106), 211-225.

Clarus, A. (1874). Ueber Aphasie bei Kinder. *Jahrbuch für Kinderheilkunde*, 7, 369-400.

Cramon, D. (1981). Traumatic mutism and the subsequent reorganization of speech functions. *Neuropsychologia* 19 (6), 801-805.

Dennis, M. (1980). Strokes in childhood: Communicative intent, expression, and comprehension after left hemisphere arteriopathy in a right-handed nine year old. In: R. W. Richer (Ed.), Language development and aphasia in children (pp. 45 - 67). New York: *Academic Press.*

Dennis, M. (2010). Language disorders in children with central nervous system Injury. *J Clin Exp Neuropsychol.* 32(4), 417-432.

Dennis, M. & Barnes, M.A. (1990). Knowing the Meaning, Getting the Point, Bridging the Gap, and Carrying the Message: Aspects of Discourse following Closed Head Injury in Childhood and Adolescence. *Brain and Language* (39), 428-446.

Dennis, M. & Levin, H.S. (2004). New perspectives on cognitive and behavioral outcome after childhood closed head injury. *Dev Neuropsychol.* (25), 1-3.

Eisenson J., & Ingram, D. (1972). Childhood aphasia: an updated concept based on recent research. *Acta Symbolica,* 3, 108-116.

Fabbro, F. (2004). Neurogenic language disorders in children. Amsterdam: *Elsevier.*

Franke, U. (2004). Logopädisches Handlexikon. München: *E. Reinhardt.*

Freud, S. (1897). Die infantile Cerebrallähmung. Wien: *Alfred Höldder.*

Friederici, A. D. (1984). Neuropsychologie der Sprache. Stuttgart: *Verlag W. Kohlhammer.*

Girolami-Boulinier, A. (1986). Die schulische Entwicklung von Kindern und Jugendlichen mit Aphasiesyndrom. In: R. Becker, & W. Elstner (Eds.), Das aphasische Kind (pp. 69-85). Berlin: *VEB Verlag Volk und Gesundheit.*

Gloning, K., & Hift, E. (1979). Beitrag zur Therapie der erworbenen Aphasie bei Kindern im Vorschulalter. In: G. Peuser (Ed.), Studien zur Sprachtherapie (pp. 235-239). München: *Wilhelm Fink Verlag.*

Goodglass, H. (1980). Disorders of naming following brain injury. *American Scientist,* 68, 647-655.

Goodglass, H., & Kaplan, E. (1972). The assessment of Aphasia and related disorders. Philadelphia: *Lea and Febiger.*

Grimm, H. (2003). Störungen der Sprachentwicklung. Göttingen: *Hogrefe.*

Guttmann, E. (1942). Aphasia in children, *Brain,* 65, 205-19.

Hahn, K., Böhringer, K., & Ritthaler, C. (2002). Fallbeispiel Timo. In: M. Loew, & K. Böhringer (Eds.), Kindliche Aphasie. Beiträge zur neurologischen Rehabilitation von Kindern, Jugendlichen und jungen Erwachsenen (pp. 45-59). Gailingen: *Hegau-Jugendwerk.*

Haynes, C. (1986). Current Therapy for Aphasic Children in Britain. In: R. Becker, & W. Elstner (Eds.), Das aphasische Kind (pp. 100-111). Berlin: *nes.*

Hécaen, H. (1976). Acquired Aphasia in Children and the Ontogenesis of Hemispheric Functional Specialization. *Brain and Language*, 3, 114-134.

Hécaen, H. (1983). Acquired aphasia in children: Revisited. *Neuropsychologia,* 21, 581-587.

Herzberg, B., & Herzberg, L. (1977). Brain damage and abnormal behaviour in children. *Med. J Aust.,* 1 (23), 853-855.

Hofmann-Stocker, E. (1991). Zur schulisch-beruflichen Entwicklung junger Aphasiker. Ergebnisse einer katamnestischen Studie. *Die Rehabilitation,* 30, 116-124.

Holland, A.L. (1970). Case studies in aphasia rehabilitation using programmed instruction. *Journal of Speech and Hearing Disorders,* 35, 377-390.

Huber, W., Poeck, K., & Weniger, D. (1997). Aphasie. In: W. Hartje, & K. Poeck (Eds.), Klinische Neuropsychologie (pp. 80 - 143). Stuttgart: *Thieme.*

Jordan, F. M., & Murdoch, B.E. (1994). Severe closed-head injury in childhood: linguistic outcomes into adulthood. *Brain Inj.,* 8, 501-508.

Jordan, F. M., & Ashton, R. (1996). Language performance of severely closed-head injured children. *Brain Inj.,* 10, 91-97.

Kubandt, M. (2008a). Aphasie bei Kindern - Einführung und Ausblick. *Die Sprachheilarbeit,* 4, 202-210.

Kubandt, M. (2008b). "Welche Schule ist die richtige für mein Kind?" - Nachsorge von Kindern mit Aphasie am Beispiel der Beschulung. In: A. Ebert, W. Fries, & L. Ludwig (Eds.), Rehabilitation und Nachsorge nach Schädelhirnverletzung (pp. 131-138). Göttingen: *Hippocampus Verlag.*

Kubandt, M. (2009). Aphasie bei Kindern und Jugendlichen. Ein Ratgeber für therapeutische Berufsgruppen. Idstein: *Schulz-Kirchner Verlag.*

Kubandt, M., & Friede, S. (2011). Diagnostik der Aphasie bei Kindern und Jugendlichen – Überblick, Möglichkeiten und Grenzen. *Forum Logopädie*, Heft 6, 25, 18-25.

Leheckovä, H. (2004). Recovery from Aphasia after Polytrauma in a Czech Child: What is lost and what is left. In: F. Fabbro (Ed.), Neurogenic language disorders in children (pp. 199-229). Amsterdam: *Elsevier.*

Leischner, A. (1987). Aphasien und Sprachentwicklungsstörungen. New York: *Thieme.*

Lenneberg, E. H. (1967). Biological foundations of language. New York: *Wiley.*

Lenneberg, E. H. (1972). On explaining language. In: M.E.P. Seligman, & J.L. Hager (Eds.), Biological boundaries of learning (pp. 379-396). New York: *Appleton-Century-Crofts.*

Loew, M., & Böhringer, K. (2002). Kindliche Aphasie. Beiträge zur neurologischen Rehabilitation von Kindern, Jugendlichen und jungen Erwachsenen. Gailingen: *Schriftreihe Jugendwerk.*

Lohmann, H., Müller-Ehrenberg, S., Deppe, S., & Knecht, S. (2005). Language lateralisation in young children assessed by functional transcranial doppler sonography. *NeuroImage,* 3, 780-790.

Loonen, M. C., & Van Dongen, H.R. (1990). Acquired childhood aphasia: Outcome one year after onset. *Archives of Neurology*, 47, 1324-1328.

Mantovani, J. F., & Landau, W. M. (1980). Acquired aphasia with convulsive disorder : course and prognosis. *Neurology*, 30, 524-529.

Martins, I. P., & Ferro, J.M. (1991). Recovery from aphasia and lesion size in the temporal lobe. In: A. P. Martins, A. Castro-Caldas, H.R. Van Dongen, & A. Van Hout (Eds.), Acquired Aphasia in Children. *Acquisition and Breakdown of Language in the Developing Brain* (pp. 171 - 184). Dordrecht: *nes.*

Martins, I.P. (2004). Persistent acquired childhood aphasia. In: F. Fabbro (Ed.), Neurogenic language disorders in children (pp. 231-251). Amsterdam: *Elsevier.*

Miller, J.F., Campbell, T.F., Chapman, R.S., & Weismer, S.E. (1984). Language Behavior in Acquired Childhood Aphasia. In: A. Holland (Ed.), Language Disorders in Children (pp. 57 - 99). San Diego: *College Hill Press.*

Niedergall, G., & Remschmidt, H. (1981). Entwicklung des Sprechens und der Sprache. In: H. Remschmidt (Ed.), Neuropsychologie des Kinderalters (pp. 148 - 168). Stuttgart: *Enke.*

Paquier, P.F., Dongen, H.R. van, Creten, W., & Borsel, J. van (1998). The fluency/nonfluency dichotomy in the spontaneous speech of children with acquired aphasia. *Acta Neurologica Belgica,* 98, 242.

Paquier, P.F., Dongen, H.R. van (1993). Current trends in acquired childhood aphasia: An introduction. *Aphasiology,* 1993, 421-440.

Paquier, P., Van Dongen, H.R. (1996). Review of research on the clinical presentation of acquired childhood aphasia. *Acta Neurologica Scandinavica,* 93, 428-36.

Paquier, P.F., Van Maldeghem, V.R., Van Dongen, H. R., & Creten, W. L. (2004). Recognizable Spontaneous Language Characteristics in a Young Adult Twelve Years after she became aphasic as a Child. In: F. Fabbro (Ed.), Neurogenic language disorders in children (pp. 181-197). Amsterdam: *Elsevier.*

Poeck, K., & Hacke, W. (2006). Neurologie. Vol 12. Berlin-Heidelberg-New York: *Springer.*

Roberts, A.C. (1966). The aphasic Child. Springfield: *Charles C. Thomas.*

Rothenberger, A. (1986). Aphasie bei Kindern. *Fortschr. Neurol. Psychiatr.,* 54, 92-98.

Rother, A. (2005). Kindliche Aphasien. *LOGOS Interdisziplinär,* 2, 90-92.

Rüttiger, L., Braun, D., Gegenfutter, K.R., Petersen, D., Schönle, D., & Sharpe L.T. (1999). Selective colour constancy deficits after circumscribed unlilateral brain lesions. *J. Neurosci,* 19, 3094-3106.

Rupp, K. (2006). Die erworbene Aphasie im Kindesalter. Eine katamnestische Untersuchung. Magisterarbeit. Bielefeld: *nes.*

Siegmüller, J., & Heide, J. (2006). Erworbene Sprachstörungen bei Kindern. In: J. Siegmüller, & H. Bartels (Eds.), Leitfaden Sprache, Sprechen, Stimme, Schlucken (pp. 266 - 282). München: *Elsevier.*

Satz, P., & Bullard-Bates, C. (1986). Acquired Aphasia in Children. In: E. Sarno (Ed.), Acquired Aphasia (pp. 399 - 426). New York: *Thieme.*

Satz, P., & Lewis, R. (1993). Acquired Aphasia in Children. In: G. Blanken, J. Dittmann, H. Grimm, J.C. Marshall, & C.-W. Wallesch (Eds.), Linguistic Disorder and Pathologies. *An international Handbook* (pp. 646 - 659). Berlin: *Walter de Gruyter.*

Schröder, G. (2003). Aufgaben der Neuropädagogik. Schulische Belastungserprobung und Integration. Seminarbericht "Neurologische Rehabilitation von Kindern und Jugendlichen" 07.-09.10.2003, Bremen: *Friedehorst.*

Sollee, N.D., & Kindlon, D.J. (1987). Lateralized brain injury and behaviour problems in children. *Abnormal Child Psychology,* 15, 479-491.

Spencer, P.G. (2006). Kindliche Aphasie. Hintergründe und Praxis. *Not*, 3, 24-26.

Spencer, P.G., & Möhrle, C. (2007). Kinder und Jugendliche mit Aphasie. *Forum Logopädie*, 6, 6-12.

Tartter, V.C. (1998). Language and it's normal processing. London: *Sage Publications.*

Tesak, J. (2001). Geschichte der Aphasie. Idstein: *Schulz-Kirchner.*

Van Dongen, H.R., & Visch-Brink, E. (1988). Naming in aphasic children of paraphasie errors. *Neuropsychologia,* 26, 629-632.

Von Dongen, H.R., & Loonen, M.C.B. (1977). Factors related to prognosis of acquired fluent aphasia in children. *Annals of Neurology,* 17, 131 136.

Van Dongen, H., Paquier, P., Creten, W., Borsel, J., & Catsman-Berrevoets, C. (2001). Clinical evaluation of conversational speech fluency in the acute phase of acquired childhood aphasia: Does a fluency/nonfluency dichotomy exist?. *Journal of Child Neurology,* 16, 345–351.

Van Hout, A., & Seron, X. (1983). L'aphasie de I'enfant. Bruxelles: *Mardaga.*

Van Hout, A., Evrard, P., & Lyon, G. (1985). On the positive semiology of acquired aphasia in children. *Developmental Medicine and Child Neurology,* 27, 231-241.

Van Hout, A. (1992). Acquired Aphasia in Children. In: S.J. Segalowitz, & I. Rapin (Eds.), Handbook of Neuropsychology (Band 7, pp. 281 - 303). Amsterdam: *Elsevier.*

Van Hout, A. (1992). Acquired aphasia in children. In: S.J. Segalowitz, & I. Rapin (Eds.), Handbook of neuropsychology: Child neuropsychology (Vol. 7., pp. 139 - 161). Amsterdam: *Elsevier.*

Van Hout, A., Martins, I.P., Castro-Caldas, A., & Dongen, H.R. van (1991). Acquired aphasia in children: Acquisition and breakdown of language in the developing brain. Dordrecht: *Kluwer.*

Visch-Brink, E.G., & Van de Sandt-koenderman, M. (1984). The occurrence of paraphasias in the spontaneous speech of children with acquired aphasia. *Brain and Language,* 23, 258-271.

In: Aphasia
Editor: Christina T. Rogers
ISBN: 978-1-63483-993-8

Chapter 3

APHASIA IN CHILDREN AND ITS IMPACT ON QUALITY OF LIFE

Michitaka Funayama, MD
Department of Neuropsychiatry, Ashikaga Red Cross Hospital
Asuka Nakajima, MSc, RST
Department of Rehabilitation, Ashikaga Red Cross Hospital, Japan

ABSTRACT

People who develop aphasia must adjust their lifestyle and learn to cope with the activity limitations that result from their disability. Aphasia can profoundly affect a person's capacity for academic achievement as well as their occupational competency, social participation, and ability to manage finances. This is especially true for young people, who have yet to fully learn how to participate as a member of society. Young people who acquire aphasia are likely to have a poor record at school and have difficulties completing higher education and getting a job. They also might be unable to pass a written test for a driver's license. Young people with aphasia who wish to contribute to the community and be engaged in social activities might not achieve these goals and might feel isolated. In the worst case, they might shut other people out of their lives and withdraw from society. In this chapter, we describe the long-term prognosis of three individuals who became aphasic in their childhood or youth and discuss how young people with aphasia can best be rehabilitated.

1. INTRODUCTION

The first verse in the Gospel of John reads, "In the beginning was the Word, and the Word was with God, and the Word was God." It is quite difficult to live without the Word. Language ability is usually taken for granted—until it is lost. Brain damage can cause aphasia and affect a wide range of language abilities including the understanding of speech, talking, reading, and writing. One can have an experience close to aphasia when visiting a foreign country where one is unable to understand others' language and unable to converse with others. However, aphasia differs from this scenario because a person with aphasia also experiences difficulty in thinking in their own language.

Aphasia can result from any type of brain damage, including stroke, traumatic brain injury, brain tumor, and infection. Approximately 30% of first-ever ischemic stroke survivors have aphasia (Engelter et al., 2006). For the person with aphasia, sudden changes in language processing immediately impact daily communication and change the nature of communicative exchanges and the quality of interactions. Although people with aphasia want to function as they have in the past, they often are unable to work and are confronted with an enormous challenge to fulfill their roles in daily living—for example as a partner, parent, or friend. Some might even develop depression (Astrome et al., 1993), which often is related to loneliness, isolation, low self-esteem, and the inability to accept themselves as a handicapped person.

Although aphasia occurs most commonly in the latter half of life, some individuals may acquire aphasia in childhood. In these cases, aphasia greatly affects the whole life.

Despite the challenges that they face, people with aphasia generally wish to be engaged, involved, and respected, to take part in the community, to be cognizant of current events, to do things with others without being a burden, to contribute to the community, and to generally carry out a daily routine. In this chapter, we describe three young people with aphasia and review the impact of aphasia on these individuals. We also discuss how to rehabilitate children with aphasia.

2. Case Presentation

Case Presentation 1

Case 1 was a 17-year-old high school student when he experienced a brain hemorrhage attributable to arteriovenous malformation. He was admitted to a hospital in his town with disturbance of consciousness. Computed tomography revealed the location of the lesion in the left temporal lobe which covered Wernicke's area and its underlying white matter, the arcuate fasciculus, which both play a critical role in linguistic functions. Surgical resection improved the disturbance of consciousness, but aphasia remained.

The aphasia was classified moderate-severity Wernicke's aphasia with poor auditory processing, fluent speech, and poor repetition. Owing to poor auditory processing, the patient had difficulty understanding others' speech. Although he spoke fluently in sentences, the content of those sentences sometimes contained verbal paraphasias as well as phonological paraphasias. Repetition was limited to a few phrases. An intensive aphasia treatment program was provided in the hospital, and the Wernicke's aphasia improved to some extent. After treatment, however, the patient still had difficulties understanding long sentences, talking, sending text messages, and learning. In contrast, he had relatively intact nonlinguistic cognitive skills, such as memory and visuospatial function.

Prior to his hemorrhage, the patient had an average school record and was a polite and friendly young man. However, he could no longer participate in the things he enjoyed such as studying at school, talking with friends, and sending text messages to friends. He was unable to pass a written driver's test and therefore could not obtain a driver's license. He gradually began to lose contact with friends and spent more time indoors enjoying computer games or reading cartoons. After graduating high school, even though he tried to work in several factories, he quit each job after a short time because he was not able to communicate well with others. He could not fully manage his finances. At 9 years post-onset, case 1 has become socially isolated.

Case Presentation 2

Case 2 was an 18-year-old high school student when he was riding his bicycle home from school and was struck by a truck. In the hospital, he was in a deep coma (Glasgow Coma Scale score 5; E1V1M3). He was intubated and mechanically ventilated. Brain computed tomography revealed left fronto-temporo-parietal hemorrhagic contusions with midline shift, which required hematoma resection as well as internal and external decompression. After 10 weeks, the patient regained consciousness and participated in neurologic rehabilitation therapy. After 6 months of therapy, he was discharged with right complete hemiparesis, total aphasia, severe apathy, and attentional dysfunction. His follow-up computed tomography at 1-year post-onset revealed brain damage that covered almost all of the left hemisphere.

The patient had global aphasia, presenting with impairment of all productive and receptive linguistic functions, which was resistant to intensive speech therapy provided in the hospital. He was unable to produce any spontaneous speech. Repetition was also totally impaired in that he could not repeat even one word. Comprehension was poor even on a word level, and he was unable to understand sentences. Comprehension of written language was also severely impaired. Communication was partly possible with the aid of non-verbal gestures. He was totally unable to manage his finances.

In summary, the communication capabilities of case 2 were extremely poor and were limited to very simple words and non-verbal gestures. The patient dropped out of high school and could not get a driver's license. He was incapable of meaningful social engagement and thus gradually lost contact with friends and often stayed indoors. Seizure control was difficult, and in the 10 years following the injury the patient had to be hospitalized several times owing to status epilepticus. At 10 years post-onset, the patient's activities were limited to going to rehabilitation four times per week for physical and linguistic improvement.

Case Presentation 3

Case 3 was a 13-year-old junior high school student when he fell from a height of 6 meters. He was in a deep coma when he arrived at the emergency department of our hospital. His traumatic brain injuries required internal and external decompression. His coma subsided, and he was discharged at 6 months post-onset. Follow-up computed tomography performed at 1-year post-onset showed damage of the left temporo-parietal cortices and the right temporal pole.

The patient had moderate-severity Wernicke's aphasia. He also presented with attentional dysfunction and executive dysfunction. Although he returned to school at 1-year post-onset, his performance was substantially poorer than his pre-accident level. He could not fully understand what his teachers were saying. His ability to perform mathematical calculations was severely compromised, and he was no longer able to perform simple additions of one figure that included carrying. He could not write some Kanji characters (Chinese characters) that are taught in the lower grades of primary school. He moved from a regular class into a special education class for handicapped children. After graduating junior high school, he entered a special support school for handicapped children where he was taught manufacturing technology, and he now hopes to get a job in a small workshop. He is unlikely to obtain driver's license because of his aphasia and attentional dysfunction.

Summary of the Three Young People with Aphasia

All three cases experienced problems with learning, vocation, driving, social communication, and making friends. Participating in society and making an optimal choice regarding vocation were the most substantive challenges during their rehabilitation.

3. Impact of Aphasia on Daily Living

Aphasia negatively affects a wide range of activities, including classroom participation, vocation, driving, social participation, and managing finances.

A. Classroom Participation

As exemplified in the case presentations above, when children with aphasia return to school, they find it difficult to learn because, for almost all subjects, learning requires linguistic abilities. Children with aphasia achieve much less than expected, and their record at school is poor relative to pre-aphasia levels.

Very often, the problems observed in the classroom setting also include difficulties with interpersonal relationships. Those patients who are overly sensitive may interpret pressure, teasing, or joking as personal attacks. Children with aphasia are likely to have fewer chances to have a boy/girlfriend. Sometimes, they are encouraged to move from a regular class into a special education class or a special support school for handicapped children.

B. Vocation

Most people with aphasia stop working shortly after aphasia onset. However, the long-term employment status of children with aphasia has not been studied. Nonetheless, several studies have addressed long-term employment status of adults with aphasia. Parr et al., (1997) studied vocational problems of 50 adults with chronic aphasia. All subjects were aged 26–92 years and were 5–15 years post-onset. The employment rate was approximately 15%, and only one of those working had returned to a level of productivity equivalent to that of pre-aphasia employment. Hinkley et al., (1998) found that, of 31 participants with stroke-induced chronic aphasia between the ages of 23 and 69 years, all of whom had been employed at the time of stroke, only 26% had returned to some level of employment, and none exhibited pre-stroke productivity. Thus, only a limited proportion of adults with aphasia seem to be able to work.

The severity of aphasia does not necessarily relate to return to work (Hinkley et al., 2002). In addition to the severity of aphasia, factors that contribute to good vocational outcome include workplace flexibility, social support, motivation, level of cognition, and level of motor impairment (Hinkley et al., 2002). Demographic factors such as age, gender, and education might also influence the ability to return to work, although these factors have not been sufficiently addressed. The Hinkley et al., (1998) study suggests that, in addition to the challenges associated with the severity of aphasia, both psychosocial issues and physical/neuropsychological functions play a critical role in a patient's ability to return to work.

Adults with aphasia who return to work with their previous employer often perform simpler types of work, whereas others have to change job because the previous job was simply too demanding. The most common difficulties in returning to work were related to job status and unwillingness to accept a position of lesser prestige even if it was necessitated by their disabilities.

There is an additional vocation-related problem for children with aphasia, and it relates to making a vocational choice. Vocational tests often require linguistic abilities and are therefore challenging for young people with aphasia. However, these young people often do not accept the more menial types of jobs suggested on the basis of vocational testing and might resent their family's efforts in arranging these jobs. Psychological and psychosocial issues should be carefully addressed before making a vocational choice.

C. Driving

Driving is a big issue for children with aphasia. In Japan, adults with aphasia who had already obtained a driver's license prior to their illness are required to get a doctor's permission to resume driving. They are able to resume driving when they are at a very low risk of seizures, have no visual or visuospatial problems, and have no attention dysfunction. Resuming driving is an important part of recovery. However, young people with aphasia have to pass a written exam to obtain their driver's license, which is highly challenging. For people with aphasia who do not drive, other transportation might also be difficult because of the requirement of buying a ticket, making a transfer, or following instructions.

D. Social Participation

People with aphasia tend to withdraw from interpersonal relationships and have small social networks. They are unable to take part in a conversation because they miss information or do not understand what has been said. Some affected individuals report a lack of symmetry in communication, and conversations tend to be one sided. Often, people with aphasia take a passive and predominantly listening role in group interactions and conversations. They feel alone even though they are with other people. Some people with aphasia feel they are a burden to others and therefore stop participating in social activities.

For most people with aphasia, the number of friends decreases after the onset of aphasia. Friends stay away because they do not know how to communicate with affected individuals, and as time passes it becomes more difficult for such individuals to make contact with others. Furthermore, making new friends is quite challenging. According to Hilari et al., 2006, 30% of people with aphasia indicated that they had no friends at 1 year or more post-onset of aphasia. Davidson et al., (2008) studied this issue by observing how many people communicated with patients during the 240 hours of observation period. They reported that people with aphasia (n = 15) communicated with only 3 strangers and with 111 acquaintances, whereas age-matched people without aphasia (n = 15) communicated with 21 strangers and 220 acquaintances. None of the people with aphasia visited friends during the observation period, whereas the age-matched people without aphasia visited a variety of places. Typical communications for people with aphasia included greeting friends at a stroke group meeting or respite center and brief conversations with friends who visited the affected individual's home, whereas typical communications for people without aphasia included extended discussions with friends and visiting and conversing with friends in their homes.

It can often be valuable to meet others with aphasia at an aphasia group. This can give persons with aphasia a sense of solidarity and make them aware that they are not alone in their affliction.

E. Managing Finances

Persons with aphasia are often unable to manage their finances independently and need assistance in budgeting. Some even require complete supervision of their funds and can sometimes express extreme frustration concerning their inability to be more involved in financial arrangements. People with aphasia often are eligible to receive a national pension in Japan; however, they may be unable to follow the procedures required to obtain this. For adults who became aphasic in childhood, managing finances can be quite difficult because most had not had any substantive experience with finances prior to the onset of aphasia.

4. REHABILITATION

Linguistic rehabilitation is provided by speech therapists. Unlike physical rehabilitation, aphasia continues to improve for many years after onset. This is especially true for young people with aphasia, some of who might experience improvement for more than a decade. The optimal rehabilitation strategy varies from person to person depending on the type of linguistic dysfunctions that are present, e.g., apraxia of speech, dysprosody, phonological impairments, and comprehension deficits. Rehabilitation aims to help patients regain communicative function to participate in activities of daily living.

A. Communication Methods

In cases of severe aphasia, communication can be accomplished nonverbally, e.g., by drawing, facial expressions, head shaking, nodding, laughter, crying, counting on fingers, pointing with hands, and gestures including rudimentary pantomime. Simple visual analog rating scales are useful to obtain information about how the person with aphasia is feeling, e.g., presenting the patient with 10 faces with expressions ranging from unhappy (1) to happy (10) and asking them to choose a face (Davidson et al., 2006). Making use of communication books or cards in which personal information is included can also facilitate conversation.

B. Communication Partners

Some caregivers have limited knowledge of aphasia whereas others have the skills required for effective communication with aphasia patients. Family members can greatly influence a patient's progress in rehabilitation. Some family members have the tendency to overprotect, excluding the aphasic individual from making decisions, whereas others are successful at promoting the individual's abilities. Family members and friends often do not know how to communicate with people with aphasia, and thus they must depend on a speech therapist to act as a bridge between patients and family members/ friends.

Typical communication skills that are effective when communicating with people with aphasia include asking closed questions, taking a speaking pause when needed, and using short sentences. If an individual with aphasia lives with people who have the knowledge and skills to adapt to the communicative limitations of the affected individual, they have a better chance of achieving social engagement.

C. Personal Factors

Physical and neuropsychological factors affect the rehabilitation process. Some people with aphasia are confronted with physical impairments that restrict their ability to engage in routine activities. These impairments may include palsy, chronic pain, poor balance, epilepsy, and fatigue. Neuropsychological factors that can affect rehabilitation include apathy, executive dysfunctions, and deficits in memory, attention span, and concentration. The more severe or numerous these conditions, the less the patient will be able to communicate socially. However, people with aphasia, even severe aphasia, can engage in activities that involve predominantly nonverbal functions, such as playing cards, drawing pictures, taking photos, and gardening, and can playing sports—if they have no palsy. These activities increase the sense of feeling connected with others.

D. How to Rehabilitate Young People with Aphasia

Young people have yet to fully learn how to participate as a member of society. Aphasia can profoundly affect their capacity for academic achievement, their future occupation, their social participation, and their home life, and they tend to withdraw from social situations.

The goal of rehabilitation for children with aphasia is to encourage them to socialize. To make the optimal vocational choice, care should be taken to ensure that they will be able to continue the chosen work. Engaging in any activities that require social participation is recommended. It is desirable that children with aphasia keep in touch with old friends. Speech therapists, family members, and communication partners are able to increase the opportunities for children with aphasia to achieve social engagement. For example, a speech therapist and a homeroom teacher in school could discuss the abilities of a child with aphasia to properly assess what he or she will be able to accomplish as a worker. This will make a positive difference in the affected child's life.

References

Astrom, M., Adolfsson, R, Asplund, K. (1993). Major depression in stroke patients. A 3-year longitudinal study. *Stroke* 24, 976-982.

Davidson, B., Howe, T., Worrall, L., Hickson, L., Togher, L. (2008). Social participation for older people with aphasia: The impact of communication disability on friendships. *Top Stroke Rehabilitation* 15, 325-340.

Davidson, B., Worrall, L., Hickson, L. (2006). Social communication in older age: Lessons from people with aphasia. *Top Stroke Rehabilitation* 13, 1-13.

Engelter, S.T., Gostynski, M., Papa, S., Frei, M., Born, C., Ajdacic-Gross, V., Gutzwiller, F., Lyrer, P.A. (2006). Epidemiology of aphasia attributable to first ischemic stroke. Incidence, severity, fluency, etiology, and thrombolysis. *Stroke* 37, 1379-1384.

Hilari, K., Northcott, S. (2006). Social support in people with chronic aphasia. *Aphasiology* 20, 17-36.

Hinkley, J.J. (1998). Investigating the predictors of lifestyle satisfaction among younger adults with chronic aphasia. *Aphasiology* 12, 509-518.

Hinkley, J.J. (2002). Vocational and social outcomes of adults with chronic aphasia. *Journal of Communication Disorders* 35, 543-560.

Parr, S., Byng, S., Gilpin, S., Ireland, C. (1997). Talking about aphasia. Philadelphia, PA: Open University Press.

In: Aphasia
Editor: Christina T. Rogers
ISBN: 978-1-63483-993-8

Chapter 4

SUBCORTICAL APHASIA: STILL AN ENIGMA

Lucia Iracema Zanotto de Mendonça*, MD, PhD
Neurology Division of São Paulo University School of Medicine
and São Paulo Catholic University, São Paulo, Brasil

ABSTRACT

The concept that aphasia is caused by subcortical lesions dates back to the 1970s. However, this subject is still controversial, even today. Many researchers believe that the cortex is the neural center for cognitive functions, including language, and aphasic symptoms observed after subcortical lesions may result, in fact, from functional impairment of cortical activity. In contrast, other authors have advocated a specific role of subcortical structures in language. Advancements in our understanding have resulted in a change of focus for this issue. The term subcortical aphasia encompasses cases of aphasia resulting from lesions located below the cortex, which includes lesions to the basal ganglia, thalamus, and white matter. Advancements in our understanding of the fascicles that travel over the white matter and that connect different cortical areas related to language have revealed that white matter lesions can produce various changes in language. Thus, to elucidate the role of subcortical structures in language, unique injuries to the basal ganglia and thalamus must be separated from those that affect the white matter. The aim of this chapter is to present evidence for the

* E-mail: lucia.iracema@terra.com.br; Adress: Rua André Dreifus – 264 – São Paulo – Brasil; Code area: 01252-010; Telephone number: (55) 11 – 3285-6046 and (55) 11 – 9.9931-9713.

specific involvement of the basal ganglia and thalamus in vocal production, speech, and language. Hypophonia, difficulties in speech initiation, disfluency, syntactic deficits and semantic-lexical disorders are specifically discussed. Thalamic and basal ganglia lesions seem to accompany more complex deficits of language. As the entire cortex has access to subcortical structures, even Broca's and Wernicke's areas, through cortico-subcortical loops, subcortical structures are predominantly integration structures and thus can participate in different aspects of communicative function. The participation of fronto-subcortical circuits and the integration with the posterior cerebral areas has been proposed. Subcortical structures possibly play an important evolutionary role in language acquisition by humans. Basal ganglia and the thalamus may have adapted its own *modus operandi* for speech functions. The cortico-subcortical network and the interrelationship between corticality and subcorticality should be considered to fully comprehend the function of language.

The notion that aphasia might be caused by subcortical lesions was formulated a few decades ago. Although ideas about subcortical aphasia have evolved over time, the subject remains controversial. Many researchers believe both that the cortex is the neural center for cognitive functions, including language, and that aphasic symptoms observed after subcortical lesions may result from the functional impairment of cortical activity. In contrast, other authors have argued that subcortical structures play a specific role in language.

Subcortical aphasia was initially understood as aphasia resulting from lesions located below the cortex, including lesions on the basal ganglia, thalamus, and white matter. Advancements in our understanding of the subcortical fascicles that travel over the white matter and connect different cortical areas related to language, which have arisen both from tractography [45] and from intraoperative stimulation of patients with brain tumors [23], have resulted in a change of focus with respect to this issue.

According to several studies, the presentation of subcortical aphasia is characterized by wide variability: in some cases, it is similar to classic cortical aphasia, whereas in others, it is not [42].

This variability might be partially understood if one considers that the language function requires both the participation and the interrelation (and thus, the connection) of multiple brain areas involved in phonological and semantic processing [45]. Other cognitive functions (such as executive functions) also participate in language processing. Subcortical fiber bundles connect the multiple brain areas required for verbal expression and comprehension in the context of human communication. Consequently, damage to one fiber bundle might cause disconnection and thus interfere with the language function in a manner that is not necessarily similar to that resulting from injury to the same cortical area.

As a function of the current state of knowledge and aiming to elucidate the role of subcortical structures in language, unique injuries to the basal ganglia and thalamus must be separated from those that affect the white matter. The aim of this chapter is to present evidence for the specific involvement of the basal ganglia and thalamus in vocal production, speech, and language. Because this matter has not yet been elucidated, this work's objective is to present the knowledge provided by recent studies, emphasizing the evidence that seems to provide the most promising basis for future research.

Anatomical-Functional Aspects

The subcortical structures discussed in this chapter are the striatum (composed of the caudate nucleus and the putamen), the globus pallidus and the thalamus.

The entire neocortex is connected to subcortical structures. The relationships between the subcortical structures and the cortex are highly organized, i.e., definitecortical areas project to subcortical targets, which in turn send information back to specific cortical areas [4], thus forming a cortico-subcortical circuit.

The striatum receives connections from the cortex and projects to the (internal and external) globus pallidus and the substantia nigra. Through a parallel connection to Luys' body, the globus pallidus projects to the thalamus, which through its connection to the cortex completes the circuit. This structure is known as the classic cortico-striato-pallido-thalamo-cortical loop (Figure 1).

Some of the synapses in the cortico-subcortical loop and parallel connections (substantia nigra and Luys' body) are faciltatory, whereas others are inhibitory.

Stimulation and inhibition also occur in the thalamus. The nucleus reticularis (NR) is a thin sheet of neurons that covers the anterior and lateral aspects of the thalamus. The NR receives projections from all of the cerebral cortices and their associated thalamic nuclei in a topographic manner, but it sends inhibitory output only to the thalamus [72]. The area in the NR that receives inputs from a given cortical area (which in turn receives thalamo-cortical input from a given thalamic nucleus) projects to the same thalamic nucleus. The NR is organized into sectors, including motor, limbic, sensory, visual and auditory subdivisions.

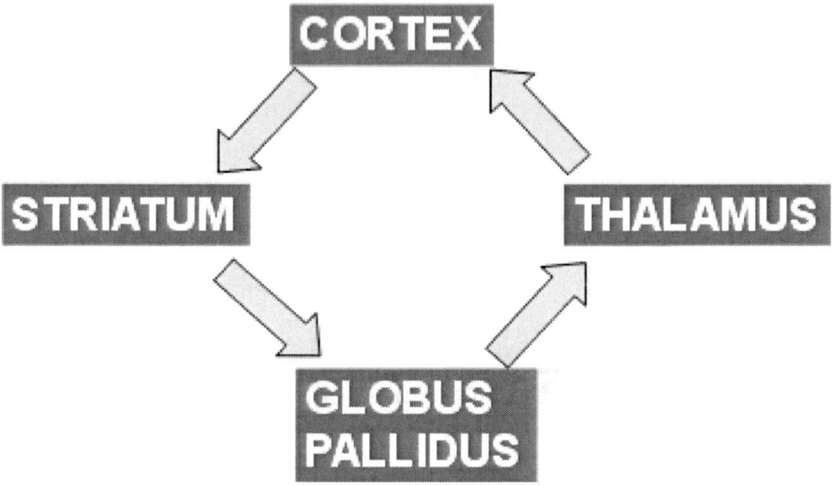

Figure 1. The cortico-striato-pallido-thalamo-cortical loop.

In other words, the signals that originate in the cortex might be reduced or amplified both along the cortico-subcortical loop and in the thalamus. The cortical information might be filtered or released in the cortico-subcortical loop; in either case, it is modified. The signals might also be modified in the thalamus, resulting in changes in the information sent to the cortex. The neurophysiological data thus indicate both that the thalamus is a center of integration and that it regulates the flow of information in the brain. Because the cortico-subcortical connections are highly organized and associated with various modalities/functions, they enable the subcortical set both to mediate communication among distinct cortical areas and to participate in the functions performed by the cortex.

The organization of the cortico-subcortical relationships might be exemplified by the case of the connections between the thalamus's medial geniculate body (MGB), which is a part of the auditory pathway, and the auditory cortex [44]. The area of the MGM that receives tonotopic inputs is connected to the primary auditory cortex, which is essentially associated with the reception of sound stimuli. In turn, the area of the MGM that receives non-tonotopic inputs is connected to secondary auditory cortical areas in which the acoustic stimuli are analyzed. Thus, the cortico-subcortical circuits could drive not only the primary cortex but also higher-order cortices.

The thalamus also includes other nuclei (Figure 2). The centromedian nucleus (CM) is an intralaminar nucleus. It is considered an extension of the brainstem reticular formation, the function of which is to activate the cortex. The thalamic nuclei that are the most involved in language disorders include the ventral anterior (VA), the ventral lateral (VL), the medial dorsal (MD) and the pulvinar (PU).

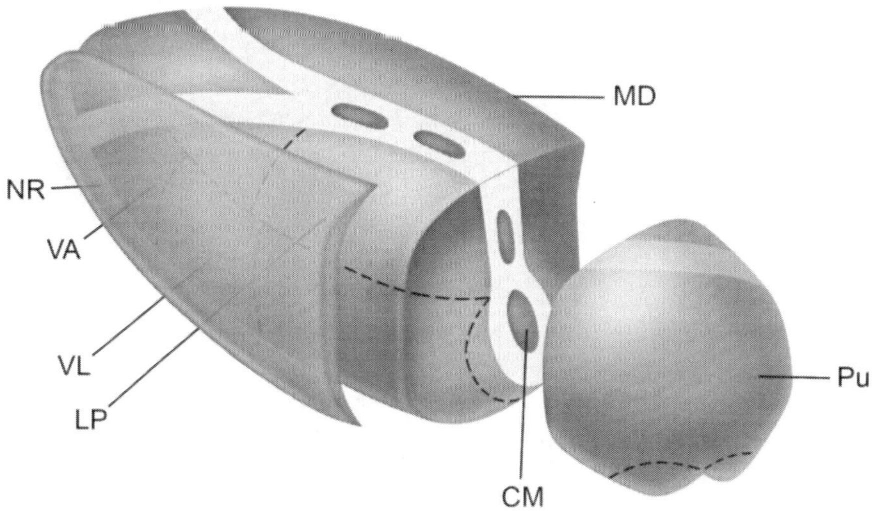

CM = centromedian nucleus; LP = lateral posterior nucleus; MD = medial dorsal nucleus; NR = nucleus reticularis; PU = pulvinar; VA = ventral anterior nucleus; VL = ventral lateral nucleus.

Figure 2. Thalamic nuclei.

Subcortical Connections of the Frontal Lobe[4]

The frontal-subcortical connections are robust and involve the cortico-striato-pallido-thalamo-cortical loop [8]. The motor and premotor cortices project to the putamen, and the premotor cortex and prefrontal cortices send information to the caudate nucleus.

The motor circuit is the frontal-subcortical circuit that encompasses the projections of the motor and premotor cortices and is related to the motor aspects of speech.

The VL nucleus of the thalamus has been associated with motor control, including speech, because it receives projections from the putamen and information from the cerebellum. Nevertheless, from the functional perspective, the VL nucleus may be subdivided into anterior, middle and posterior portions. The middle portion is more specifically related to the motor circuit. The function attributed to the other portions is described later in this chapter.

The anterior cingulum circuit is motivational, i.e., it is involved in the initiation, maintenance and sequencing of behavior, including speech. The circuits of the orbital and dorsolateral pre-frontal areas relate language to the executive functions, which are relevant for communicative behavior. The main thalamic nuclei that participate in these circuits are the VA, the VL and the MD. Although the main efference of the MD nucleus is the prefrontal cortex, in particular its dorsolateral portion, this nucleus is also connected to the cingulate gyrus, amygdala and temporal cortex [7], which is important for interaction with the emotional context during verbal communication.

Subcortical Connections of the Parietal and Temporal Lobes

The lateral posterior (LP) nucleus of the thalamus is related to the parietal cortex, whereas the pulvinar is related to all of the retro-rolandic areas and to the prefrontal cortex [36]. Together, the LP nucleus and the PU form the lateral posterior-pulvinar complex, which is the largest nucleus in the human thalamus. From the phylogenetic perspective, in humans, the development of this complex paralleled that of the parietal-temporal-occipital association cortex [58].

Subcortical Connections of Broca's and Wernicke's Areas

Recently, connections between the cortical language areas and the basal ganglia and thalamus have been demonstrated.

Direct connections from Broca's area (the pars triangularis and the pars opercularis) to the anterior putamen and to the nucleus VA of the thalamus have been mapped [24].

Strong connectivity of the thalamus, caudate nucleus and putamen/globus pallidus with Broca's and Wernicke's areas has been found. This connectivity is either bilateral and symmetric [10, 69] or lateralized to the left [10, 69].

These studies indicate the existence of a circuit that includes the basal ganglia, thalamus, and cortical language regions. Although the meaning of this circuit remains unknown, its existence is a prerequisite that substantiates its support for language processing [24].

Clinical Aspects

Overall, subcortical thalamic and non-thalamic (basal ganglia injury) aphasias exhibit the following characteristics:

1) Reversibility;
2) Speech motor production disorders: dysarthria, initiation difficulties, speed abnormalities and disfluency;
3) Repetition is often preserved [19];
4) Fluency: aphasia might be either fluent or non-fluent; and
5) Comprehension, which tends to be better preserved than expression. When comprehension is affected, faster recovery of comprehension skills is observed [42].

Differences were described in the presentation of aphasia caused by thalamic versus non-thalamic lesions.

Non-thalamic aphasia is characterized by the wider variability in its presentation. The language disorders associated with non-thalamic aphasia often correspond to those associated with classic cortical aphasia [33]. Hypophonia, i.e., reduced vocal volume, is present. Syntactic simplification of sentences is observed. Phonologic paraphasias are more common in non-thalamic than in thalamic lesions [43].

The manifestations of thalamic aphasia are considered more characteristic. The aphasias that result from anterior or posterior thalamic lesions can have striking similarities [20]. Either speech is fluent [57] or its fluency might be reduced [19] in a manner that becomes dependent on stimulation. Mutism occurs in cases with bilateral thalamic lesions. Patients can show nonfluent aphasia soon after stroke, but within a period of a few days, patients are more commonly described as having fluent output [20]. However, decreased fluency in output might continue for many months after injury [19]. Comprehension is less impaired. Comprehension might be significantly affected, especially at the phrase level, either when it includes many items or when its syntax is complex, which suggests involvement of the working memory [20]. Anomia and semantic paraphasia complete the clinical picture. At times, paraphasias are so severe as to deteriorate into jargon [20]. Lexical-semantic disorders are the most striking characteristic of thalamic aphasia [19].

Next, the pathophysiological mechanisms of some of the aforementioned clinical aspects are described and discussed.

REVERSIBILITY

In subcortical lesions, the symptoms of aphasia are of a reversible, often transient nature. The clinical manifestations might change over the course of a few days [20]. Aphasia caused by subcortical lesions tends to be less severe than aphasia caused by cortical injury. Most patients recover to a significant degree within 6 months of the ictus [29].

The prevailing concept among researchers is that the cortex is the neural center of language. Thus, the symptoms of aphasia found in cases with subcortical lesions result from cortical dysfunction. In turn, cortical reorganization allows for the recovery of the impaired function, thus accounting for the benign and transient nature of subcortical aphasias.

As a function of the relevance of the cortical-subcortical loops, mechanisms that involve diaschisis (cortical functional deafferentation) seem to account for the occurrence of cortical dysfunction. Positron emission tomography (PET) and single-photon emission computed tomography (SPECT) scans of subcortical lesions demonstrated hypometabolism/ hypoperfusion not only in the affected areas but also in the distant cortex. Some authors have found an association between the degree of cortical hypometabolism and the severity of speech disorders. Improved performance often occurs in parallel to cortical activity's return to its normal level [13].

In an elegant study using perfusion and diffusion magnetic resonance imaging (MRI), Hillis et al. [34] (2002) have demonstrated both that pure subcortical infarctions are associated with cortical hypoperfusion and that the symptoms of aphasia disappear once the cortical blood supply is restored. However, A.E. Hillis's own group admits to having observed aphasia in some cases of isolated left thalamic infarcts without cortical hypoperfusion [62].

The cause of the potential reversibility of aphasic symptoms in subcortical lesions continues to be debated.

HYPOPHONIA

Hypophonia—i.e., reduced voice intensity—is traditionally considered a characteristic of lesions that affect subcortical structures and/or their pathways. Upon request, the patient might transiently increase his or her voice volume but then reduce it again.

Little is known about the cortical areas involved in human vocalization. A functional MRI (fMRI) shows the primary sensorimotor cortex, supplementary motor area and anterior cingulum to be active [55].

The motor circuit, which is phylogenetically older, likely controls the voice volume, whereas the motivational circuit is likely involved in the initiation and maintenance of vocalization. The anterior cingulum plays an important role in vocalization in an emotional context [7]. Adjustments likely occur in the transposition of non-human to human vocalization in the course of phylogenesis.

MOTOR SPEECH DISORDERS

Dysarthria, disfluency with perseveration and changes in the rapidity of speech are found in cases that involve subcortical damage.

Dysarthria

The left putamen receives information from the motor and premotor cortices and participates in the articulation process. Stimulation of the left putamen causes anarthria [28]. The VL is the main nucleus of the thalamus associated with the motor loop.

Studies conducted with multilingual individuals, who exhibit a vast articulatory repertoire, confirm the participation of the putamen in the control of articulation. In such individuals, the activation of the left putamen increases when they speak a non-native language, but only if they are not highly proficient in that language [3]. Gray matter density is increased in the left putamen of multilinguals compared to monolinguals [3].

An affected frontal-subcortical motor circuit may cause dysarthria.

Disfluency

Occurrence of disfluency is frequently reported in cases that involve subcortical injury. Neurogenic stuttering has been associated with lesions in almost any brain area. Nevertheless, in 75% of the cases documented through neuroimaging, the lesions had a subcortical location [47] in either the basal ganglia or the cortico-subcortical circuit.

Stimulation of the middle portion of the left VL nucleus causes either perseveration on the first syllable [54] or stuttering speech [32].

Studies that are more recent suggest that the subcortical networks related to motor speech extend beyond the VL nucleus. Stuttering or syllable perseveration has been documented after CM thalamic stimulation [5], after stimulation of the internal globus pallidus [52], after combined cerebellar and thalamic lesions [64] and after stimulation of the left caudate nucleus [28]. Therefore, several thalamic nuclei, the basal ganglia and cerebellum are involved in the speech motor function.

The underlying mechanisms of disfluency in subcortical lesions remain unclear. A possible explanation for this phenomenon is that the basal ganglia play a key role in behavioral timing and sequential processing [18]. In language, the temporal sequencing process appears at most linguistic levels, from the sequencing of phonemes to form words to the sequencing of words to form a sentence to the sequencing of sentences within the context of discourse [38]. Altered sequential-processing capacity may explain the occurrence of disfluency and perseveration in the speech of patients with subcortical injury.

The relevance of the left striatum to linguistic sequencing has recently been confirmed. Participants were required either to rearrange materials sequentially based on linguistic or non-linguistic rules or to repeat a previously ordered sequence as a control task. fMRI data revealed a strongly active left-lateralized corticostriatal network that encompassed the striatum, dorsolateral and ventrolateral prefrontal cortex and presupplementary motor area while the participants were sequencing materials using linguistic versus non-linguistic rules.

Non-linguistic sequencing did not recruit this network; instead, its activation foci were both more posterior and more symmetrical. The authors suggest that the anterior striatum has extended its original sequencing role to subserve the function of linguistic sequencing in a domain-specific manner [12].

SYNTACTIC ASPECTS

Significant activation of the left caudate nucleus [50] and left putamen [25, 26] occurs during syntactic processing tasks. Although lesions in the thalamus cause difficulty both in sentence comprehension and in the use of complex syntax for verbal production [22], this difficulty may be caused by the participation of executive functioning and/or working memory, as discussed below. Syntax does not seem to require the support of thalamic processing [20].

Syntactic aspects have been relatively less studied in cases that involve subcortical lesions, particularly cases caused by vascular problems. Huntington's disease (HD) is considered a good model for the study of the participation of the basal ganglia in cognitive functions because the neuropathology at the pre-HD stage appears largely restricted to the caudate nucleus and related structures. It has been reported that Huntington's chorea is related to particular difficulties with increased grammatical complexity [35].

The findings of studies of HD patients have implicated the neostriatum in rule-governed (grammatical) aspects of language that involve both syntax and morphology [53, 65]. Teichman et al. [66] (2008) have applied three rule/lexicon tasks drawn from word morphology, syntax and a non-linguistic domain (namely, arithmetic) in early-stage HD patients. Using PET scanning, those authors have concluded that the left striatum encompasses linguistic and arithmetic circuits. In particular, the ventral area may be dedicated to rule computations.

The grammatical difficulties exhibited by patients with HD do not seem to be caused by an alteration of the working memory. The striatum seems to play a genuine role in syntactic processing that cannot be reduced to its involvement in working memory [60].

A functional cortical-subcortical syntax pathway that links Broca's area (BA45) and the left caudate head and that is associated with syntactic complexity has recently been described [67]. Those authors emphasize the functional relevance of the frontostriatal circuits and the integration of the striatum into this cortex-centered syntax network.

Semantic Aspects: Frontal-Subcortical Connections

Specific Cortical Activation and Focused Attention

The role of the intralaminar thalamic nuclei, such as the CM nucleus, in the diffuse activation of the cortex is very well known. Nevertheless, there is some evidence that the thalamus may regulate the cortical alertness and activation for a given specific function [51].

Stimulation of the left CM nucleus induces faster, more accurate responses to naming and language-comprehension tests [9]. Stimulation of the anterior portion of the VL nucleus increases speech rapidity and reduces response latency on visual naming tests [32]. Occurrence of tachylalia (increased speech speed) has been described in cases with subcortical injury.

The aforementioned data point to the participation of the activating system. By increasing the excitability of the cortical area to which it projects, this system may promote selective activation of the cortical areas needed for an ongoing function/activity. Multiple cortical areas that participate in the function in question may therefore be activated.

Nadeau and Crosson [51] (1997) have suggested the term "selective engagement" to refer to this process of temporarily engaging the topographically disparate regions of the cortex that are necessary to perform a task. Considering the proposed role of the frontal cortex in this process, the authors considered selective engagement as a form of guided attention.

Several thalamic nuclei have been described as being components of the "specific alerting system" [32], including the anterior portions of the VL, the VA, the CM, the PU and the NR nuclei.

Selective engagement appears to be accompanied by gamma rhythms (20-80 Hz) in both the cortical and the thalamic structures. Macdonald et al. [48] (1998) have shown that stimulation of an NR sector in rats induced gamma-frequency oscillations in the cortical areas associated with that region, which suggests that the NR plays a role in selective engagement. However, other thalamic nuclei might also induce rhythmic cortical activity. The possible role of the pulvinar is discussed below.

The cortico-subcortical loop is perhaps a component of the specific activating system. One study that has applied PET combined with a dopaminergic marker has found a correlation between the speed of phonological processing and left putamen activity [68].

The subcortical structures, particularly the thalamus, may optimize the allocation of focused attention for linguistic processing [49].

The hypothesis that subcortical structures participate in selective attentional processes indicates frontal-cortical connections.

Lexical Selection

Word-finding deficits are frequently found in cases that involve subcortical damage.

Stimulation of the posterior portion of the left VL nucleus and the lateral posterior-pulvinar complex causes anomia [54].

Naming is a complex task that demands the participation of several cognitive processes. In figure naming, visual recognition leads to a semantic representation of the object. The concept is then associated with an appropriate lexicon (word), which is selected among various similar options within the category to which it belongs. Once the lexicon has been selected, the individual must access the phonological representation of the word in question. These steps are interrelated and involve several brain areas.

The left prefrontal cortex is important for the lexical-semantic search and selection mechanisms. Individuals search for and retrieve (access) the lexicon in the semantic memory and select the appropriate option among many competing alternatives, which are then discarded.

Verbal fluency tests reflect this lexical search and selection. Several word generation tasks, such as verb generation [56], generating members of a semantic category and rhyme production [21], are related to the activation of the pre-supplementary motor area, cingulum, dorsal caudate, nucleus of the thalamus VA, inferior frontal gyrus and middle frontal gyrus of the dominant hemisphere. It has been found that the caudate enhances neural activity related to correct choices and suppresses activity related to incorrect choices [15, 16].

Studies of bilingualism have confirmed the relevance of the subcortical structures in the mechanisms for attention and lexical selection. Bilingual individuals need to recruit attention and selection mechanisms to control competition between their two languages. The basal ganglia play a key role in behavioral switching processing [18]. In bilingual aphasic individuals, words from both languages may appear in their verbal expression as a function of the damage to the frontal-subcortical loop [1]. In bilingual individuals, there is now evidence that the head of the left caudate, the pre-supplementary motor area and the cingulum are involved in selecting the less-proficient language when language switching [2, 27].

Therefore, the available studies indicate that the caudate nucleus and the thalamus might contribute to the process of lexical selection that occurs in the frontal cortex. Naming errors and semantic paraphasia may be the result of damage to these structures.

The frontal-subcortical circuits are becoming increasingly relevant in the study of subcortical aphasia. Subcortical lesions seem to be attended by more executive, complex language deficits [11]. In fact, some studies have noted the participation of subcortical structures in tasks that depend on the executive function, such as the elaboration of discourse and the interpretation of ambiguous or figurative passages [14, 17, 37]. Difficulties in comprehending sentences that are long and that have complex grammar may be related to the working memory [20].

Semantic Integration

Raymer et al. [59] (1997) have developed a test battery to distinguish among deficits at the purely lexical level, deficits at the purely semantic level, and deficits at the lexical-semantic interface. Those authors have applied the battery to patients with left thalamic lesions, concluding that the problem was located at the lexical-semantic interface. They have hypothesized the loss of the frontal-thalamic system's ability to selectively access the correct word.

However, another explanation is based on an inability to bind the semantic attributes that represent a concept to their corresponding lexical representation, which also results in naming errors. This hypothesis was investigated by Kraut M. A., Hart J. and colleagues [31].

Those authors have constructed a task that probes object retrieval from the integration of two features of the object. For example, "desert" and "humps" can be combined to make "camel."

fMRI has shown that successful retrievals are attended by activation of the pre-supplementary motor area, the caudate nuclei, the thalamic nuclei DM and pulvinar, and ventral temporo-occipital lobes [6, 39, 40, 41]. When object attributes were presented as word pairs, thalamic activity was limited to the left side [41]. When object features were presented in a word-picture pair, thalamic activity was bilateral [40]. Activity in the MD nucleus appeared to precede activity in the PU [39]. Those authors have hypothesized both that the earlier activity in the MD nucleus (with predominantly frontal cortex connections) was involved in a semantic search for a match and that later PU activity was involved in binding the features together in the process of object recognition.

The semantic system is widely distributed in the cortex [30]. The notion of an object derives from its visual image, the sound it produces, the motion it performs, its odor and taste and other attributes, in addition to the word that designates it. Different anterior and posterior cortical areas process the various characteristics of an object and are bound together to achieve its semantic representation.

Several lines of research have demonstrated that the PU synchronizes the neural activity of related cortical regions [31]. Slotnick et al. [63] (2002) have recorded thalamic and cortical activity during a single task of naming a target based on two attributes, detecting an increase in gamma activity at thalamic and cortical locations. Cortical and thalamic responses were phase locked, suggesting that they were related.

The PU nucleus is connected not only to the parietal, temporal and occipital cortices but also to the prefrontal cortex. The pulvinar is ideally positioned to achieve the functional integration of geographically separate but semantically related areas [31, 32, 70], thus uniting various elements to achieve the semantic representation of an object.

That hypothesis does not exclude either the lexical search and selection mechanisms or the role of the frontal-subcortical connections. However, it includes a mechanism of integration between the anterior and posterior areas for the purpose of semantic representation. This model agrees with the findings reported by Raymer et al. [59] (1997), which indicates that thalamic lesions are associated with a deficit at the lexical-semantic interface. In addition, this hypothesis accounts for the clinical manifestations of aphasia due to thalamic injury, in which the main alteration has a lexical semantic nature and is characterized by anomia and semantic paraphasia.

The participation of the basal ganglia in that model cannot be ruled out, although according to some authors [70], they do not play a role. Lexical-semantic difficulties are found in patients subjected to pallidotomy [71]. Some studies suggest that the striatum is involved in the stage of language processing during which the syntactic-semantic-contextual set is analyzed, i.e., when the appropriate response is selected according to the given context [46]. This late-stage integration takes place after the first lexical access and reflects processing at the sentence level in a given context, i.e., when semantic representation is allied both to the communicative situation and to the grammatical structure.

Based on the current state of knowledge, we can affirm that there is some evidence that the subcortical structures participate in the lexical-semantic mechanisms in harmony with the cortex.

Final Considerations

Despite the advances in research and neurophysiological and neuroimaging techniques, we still lack an understanding of the role played by basal ganglia and the thalamus in language. More specifically, the role of the striatum remains controversial.

Clinical practice and research studies indicate that the aforementioned structures participate not only in vocalization and the motor aspects of speech but also in syntactic and lexical-semantic processing.

The primary controversy is between researchers who believe that the symptoms of aphasia associated with subcortical lesions are actually caused by cortical dysfunction and researchers who believe that subcortical structures play a specific role in both language and speech.

Nevertheless, instead of independence, it seems more reasonable to posit an interrelationship between the cortex and subcortical structures. The basal ganglia and the thalamus participate in mechanisms involved in activating and regulating the cortical processing of language and speech.

Any view of the role played by the subcortical structures in cognitive functions should consider the evolution of the nervous system, which occurred as a hierarchical process, compared to the evolution of the most recent structures, whose functions developed over the functions of the oldest structure. In human ontogenesis, the brain maturation process results in the increasing relevance, during adolescence, of cortical regions in commanding the global network, whereas the caudate, cerebellum, thalamus, fusiform and parahippocampal gyri lose their relevance [61]. An older area might adjust to a newer function, not by specifically participating in it but by using its own *modus operandi* to support it. For example, the hesitancy, perseveration in the first syllable and disfluency that manifest in the speech of patients with subcortical lesions may be part of the general problem of initiating and sequencing any movement [8].

Therefore, it is possible that the basal ganglia and the thalamus do not have a specifically linguistic function. However, in the course of evolution they may have adapted a canonical circuitry for speech functions [8].

This subject should instigate further research. Subcortical structures might have played an important evolutionary role in humans' language acquisition. To fully comprehend the function of language, both the cortico-subcortical network and the interrelationship between corticality and subcorticality should be considered.

REFERENCES

[1] Abutalebi J; Annoni JM; Zimine I; Pegna AJ; Seghier ML; Lee-Jahnke H; Lazeyras F; Cappa SF; Khateb A (2008). Language control and lexical competition in bilinguals: an event-related FMRI study. *Cereb Cortex* 18(7):1496-505.

[2] Abutalebi J; Della Rosa PA; Ding G; Weekes B; Costa A; Green DW (2013). Language proficiency modulates the engagement of cognitive control areas in multilinguals. *Cortex* 49 (3):905-11.

[3] Abutalebi J; Della Rosa PA; Gonzaga AK; Keim R; Costa A; Perani D (2013). The role of the left putamen in multilingual language production. *Brain Lang* 125(3):307-15.

[4] Alexander GE; DeLong MR; Strick PL (1986). Parallel organization of functionally segregated circuits linking basal ganglia and cortex. *Annu Rev Neurosc* 9:357-81.

[5] Allert N; Kelm D; Blahak C; Capelle H H; Krauss J K (2010). Stuttering induced by thalamic deep brain stimulation for dystonia. *Journal of Neural Transmission* 117, 617–620.

[6] Assaf M; Calhoun V D; Kuzu C H; Kraut M A; Rivkin P R; Hart J; Pearlson GD (2006). Neural correlates of the object-recall process in semantic memory. *Psychiatry Research*, 147(2–3), 115–126.

[7] Barbas H (2000). Connections underlying the synthesis of cognition, memory, and emotion in primate prefrontal cortices. *Brain Res Bull* 52(5):319-30.

[8] Barbas H; García-Cabezas MÁ; Zikopoulos B (2013). Frontal-thalamic circuits associated with language. *Brain Lang* 126(1):49-61.

[9] Bhatnagar SC; Mandybur G T (2005). Effects of intralaminar thalamic stimulation on language functions. *Brain Lang* 92: 1–11.

[10] Broser PJ; Groeschel S; Hauser TK; Lidzba K; Wilke M (2012). Functional MRI-guided probabilistic tractography of cortico-cortical and cortico-subcortical language networks in children. *Neuroimage* 63(3):1561-70.

[11] Carrera E; Bogousslavsky J (2006). The thalamus and behavior: effects of anatomically distinct strokes. *Neurology* 66: 1817–1823.

[12] Chan SH; Ryan L; Bever TG (2013). Role of the striatum in language: Syntactic and conceptual sequencing. *Brain Lang* 125(3):283-94.

[13] Choi JY; Lee KH; Na D L; Byun HS; Lee SJ; Kim H; Kwon M; Lee KH; Kim BT (2007). Subcortical aphasia after striatocapsular infarction: quantitative analysis of brain perfusion SPECT using statistical parametric mapping and a statistical probabilistic anatomic map. *J. Nucl. Med.* 48, 194–200.

[14] Copland DA (2006). Meaning selection and the subcortex: Evidence of reduced lexical ambiguity repetition effects following subcortical lesions. *J Psycholinguist Res* 35: 51-66.

[15] Copland DA; Chenery HJ; Murdoch BE (2000). Processing lexical ambiguities in word triplets: Evidence of lexical–semantic deficits following dominant nonthalamic subcortical lesions. *Neuropsychology* 14: 379–390.

[16] Copland DA; Chenery HJ; Murdoch BE (2001). Discourse priming of homophones in individuals with dominant subcortical lesions, cortical lesions, and Parkinson's disease. *J Clin Exp Neuropsychol* 23, 338–356.

[17] Copland DA; de Zubicaray GI; McMahon K; Wilson SJ; Eastburn M; Chenery HJ (2003). Brain activity during automatic semantic priming revealed by event-related functional magnetic resonance imaging. *Neuroimage* 20(1):302-10.

[18] Coull JT; Cheng RK; Meck WH (2011). Neuroanatomical and neurochemical substrates of timing. *Neuropsychopharmacology* 36: 3–25.

[19] Cox DE; Heilman KM (2011). Dynamic-intentional thalamic aphasia: a failure of lexical-semantic self-activation. *Neurocase* 7(4):313-7.

[20] Crosson B (2013). Thalamic mechanisms in language: a reconsideration based on recent findings and concepts. *Brain Lang* 126(1):73-88.

[21] Crosson B; Benefield H; Cato MA; Sadek JR; Moore AB; Wierenga CE; Gopinath K; Soltysik D; Bauer RM; Auerbach EJ; Gökçay D; Leonard CM; Briggs RW (2003). Left and right basal ganglia and frontal activity during language generation: Contributions to lexical, semantic, and phonological processes. *J Int Neuropsychol Soc* 9(7): 1061–1077.

[22] De Witte L; Wilssens I; Engelborghs S; De Deyn PP; Mariën P (2006). Impairment of syntax and lexical semantics in a patient with bilateral paramedian thalamic infarction. *Brain Lang* 96(1):69-77.

[23] Duffau H; Peggy Gatignol ST; Mandonnet E; Capelle L; Taillandier L (2008). Intraoperative subcortical stimulation mapping of language pathways in a consecutive series of 115 patients with Grade II glioma in the left dominant hemisphere. *J Neurosurg* 109(3):461-71.

[24] Ford AA; Triplett W; Sudhyadhom A; Gullett J; McGregor K; Fitzgerald DB; Mareci T; White K; Crosson B (2013). Broca's area and its striatal and thalamic connections: a diffusion-MRI tractography study. *Front Neuroanat* 7:8, 2013.

[25] Friederici AD; Kotz AS (2003). The brain basis of syntactic processes: functional imaging and lesion studies. *Neuroimage* 20 Suppl 1:S8-17.

[26] Friederici AD; Kotz SA; Werheid K; Hein G; von Cramon DY (2003). Syntactic comprehension in Parkinson' disease: investigating early automatic and late integrational processes using event-related brain potentials. *Neuropsychology* 17: 133-142.

[27] Garbin G; Costa A; Sanjuan A; Forn C; Rodriguez-Pujadas A; Ventura N; Belloch V; Hernandez M; Avila C (2011). Neural bases of language switching in high and early proficient bilinguals. *Brain Lang* 119(3):129-35.

[28] Gil Robles S; Gatignol P; Capelle L; Mitchell MC; Duffau H (2005). The role of dominant striatum in language: a study using intraoperative electrical stimulations. *J Neurol Neurosurg Psychiatry* 76(7):940-6.

[29] Graff-Radford N; Eslinger P; Damasio A; Yamada T (1984). Nonhemorrhagic infarction of the thalamus: Behavioral, anatomic, and physiologic correlates. *Neurology* 34: 14–23.

[30] Hart J; Anand, R., Zoccoli, S., Maguire, M., Gamino, J., Tillman, G., et al. (2007). Neural substrates of semantic memory. *J Int Neuropsychol Soc* 13(5): 865–880.

[31] Hart J; Maguire MJ; Motes M; Mudar RA; Chiang HS; Womack KB; Kraut MA (2013). Semantic memory retrieval circuit: role of pre-SMA, caudate, and thalamus. *Brain Lang* 126(1):89-98.

[32] Hebb AO; Ojemann GA (2013). The thalamus and language revisited. *Brain Lang* 126(1):99-108.

[33] Hillis AE; Barker PB; Wityk RJ; Aldrich EM; Restrepo L; Breese EL; Work M (2004). Variability in subcortical aphasia is due to variable sites of cortical hypoperfusion. *Brain Lang* 89(3):524-30.

[34] Hillis AE; Wityk RJ; Barker PB; Beauchamp NJ; Gailloud P; Murphy K; Cooper O; Metter EJ (2002). Subcortical aphasia and neglect in acute stroke: The role of cortical hypoperfusion. *Brain* 125(Pt 5): 1094–1104.

[35] Jensen AM; Chenery HJ; Copland DA (2006). A comparison of picture description abilities in individuals with vascular subcortical lesions and Huntington's Disease. *J Commun Disord* 39(1):62-77.

[36] Jones EG (2007). The Thalamus. New York: Cambridge University Press.

[37] Ketteler D; Kastrau F; Vohn R; Huber W (2008). The subcortical role of language processing. High level linguistic features such as ambiguity-resolution and the human brain; an fMRI study. *Neuroimage* 39(4):2002-9.

[38] Kotz SA; Schwartze M; Schmidt-Kassow M (2009). Non-motor basal ganglia functions: a review and proposal for a model of sensory predictability in auditory language perception. *Cortex* 45(8):982-90.

[39] Kraut MA; Calhoun V; Pitcock JA; Cusick C; Hart J (2003). Neural hybrid model of semantic object memory: Implications from event-related timing using fMRI. *J Int Neuropsychol Soc* 9(7): 1031–1040.

[40] Kraut MA; Kremen S; Moo LR; Segal JB; Calhoun V; Hart J (2002a). Object activation in semantic memory from visual multimodal feature input. *J Cogn Neurosci* 14(1): 37–47.

[41] Kraut MA; Kremen S; Segal JB; Calhoun V; Moo LR; Hart J (2002b). Object activation from features in the semantic system. *J Cogn Neurosci* 14(1): 24–36.

[42] Krishnan G; Tiwari S; Pai AR; Rao SN (2012). Variability in aphasia following subcortical hemorrhagic lesion. *Ann Neurosci* 19(4):158-60.

[43] Kuljic-Obradovic DC (2003). Subcortical aphasia: Three different language disorder syndromes? *Eur J Neurol* 10(4): 445–448.

[44] Llano D A; Sherman S M (2008). Evidence for nonreciprocal organization of the mouse auditory thalamocortical-corticothalamic projection systems. *J Comp Neurol* 507(2): 1209–1227.

[45] Lemaire JJ; Golby A; Wells WM; Pujol S; Tie Y; Rigolo L; Yarmarkovich A; Pieper S; Westin CF; Jolesz F; Kikinis R (2013). Extended Broca's area in the functional connectome of language in adults: combined cortical and subcortical single-subject analysis using fMRI and DTI tractography. *Brain Topogr* 26(3):428-41.

[46] Longworth CE; Keenan SE; Barker RA; Marslen-Wilson WD; Tyler LK (2005). The basal ganglia and rule-governed language use: evidence from vascular and degenerative conditions. *Brain* 128(Pt 3):584-96.

[47] Ludlow C L; Loucks T (2003). Sttutering: a dynamic motor control disorder. *J Fluency Disord* 22: 273-295.

[48] Macdonald KD; Fifkova E; Jones MS; Barth DS (1998). Focal stimulation of the thalamic reticular nucleus induces focal gamma waves in cortex. *J Neurophysiol* 79(1): 474–477.

[49] McAlonan K; Cavanaugh J; Wurtz RH (2008). Guarding the gateway to cortex with attention in visual thalamus. *Nature* 456: 391–394.

[50] Moro A; Tettamanti M; Perani D; Donati C; Cappa SF; Fazio F (2001). Syntax and the brain: disentandling Grammar by selective anomalies. *Neuroimage* 13: 110-118.

[51] Nadeau SE; Crosson B (1997). Subcortical aphasia. *Brain Lang* 58(3): 355– 402; discussion 418–323.

[52] Nebel A; Reese R; Deuschl G; Mehdorn HM; Volkmann J (2009). Acquired stuttering after pallidal deep brain stimulation for dystonia. *J Neural Transm* 116: 167–169.

[53] Nemeth D; Dye CD; Sefcsik T; Janacsek K; Turi Z; Londe Z; Klivenyi P; Kincses ZT; Szabó N; Vecsei L; Ullman MT (2012). Language deficits in pre-symptomatic Huntington's disease: evidence from Hungarian. *Brain Lang* 121(3):248-53.

[54] Ojemann GA (1977). Asymmetric function of the thalamus in man. *Ann N Y Acad Sci* 299: 380–396.

[55] Olthoff A; Baudewig J; Kruse E; Dechent P (2008). Cortical sensorimotor control in vocalization: a functional magnetic resonance imaging study. *Laryngoscope* 118(11):2091-6.

[56] Petersen SE; Fox PT; Posner MI; Mintun M; Raichle ME (1988). Positron emission tomographic studies of the cortical anatomy of single-word processing. *Nature* 331(6157): 585–589.

[57] Radanovic M; Scaff M (2003). Speech and language disturbances due to subcortical lesions. *Brain Lang* 84(3): 337–352.

[58] Rakic P. (1974). Embryonic development of the pulvinar–LP complex in man. In I. S. Cooper et al. (Eds.), *The pulvinar–LP complex* (pp. 3–30). *Springfield,* IL: Thomas.

[59] Raymer AM; Moberg P; Crosson B; Nadeau S; Rothi LJ (1997). Lexicalsemantic deficits in two patients with dominant thalamic infarction. *Neuropsychologia* 35(2): 211–219.

[60] Sambin S; Teichmann M; de Diego Balaguer R; Giavazzi M; Sportiche D; Schlenker P; Bachoud-Lévi AC (2012). The role of the striatum in sentence processing: disentangling syntax from working memory in Huntington's disease. *Neuropsychologi*a 50(11):2625-35.

[61] Sato JR; Salum GA; Gadelha A; Vieira G; Zugman A; Picon FA; Pan PM; Hoexter MQ; Anés M; Moura LM; Del'Aquilla MA; Crossley N;

Amaro Junior E; Mcguire P; Lacerda AL; Rohde LA; Miguel EC; Jackowski AP; Bressan RA (2015). Decreased centrality of subcortical regions during the transition to adolescence: a functional connectivity study. *Neuroimage* 104:44-51.

[62] Sebastian R; Schein MG; Davis C; Gomez Y; Newhart M; Oishi K; Hillis AE (2014). Aphasia or Neglect after Thalamic Stroke: The Various Ways They may be Related to Cortical Hypoperfusion. *Front Neurol* 5:231.

[63] Simard F; Monetta L; Nagano-Saito A; Monchi O (2013). A new lexical card-sorting task for studying fronto-striatal contribution to processing language rules. *Brain Lang* 125(3):295-306.

[64] Slotnick SD; Moo LR; Kraut MA; Lesser RP; Hart J (2002). Interactions between thalamic and cortical rhythms during semantic memory recall in human. *Proc Natl Acad Sci USA* 99(9): 6440–6443.

[65] Tani T; Sakai Y (2010). Stuttering after right cerebellar infarction: A case study. *J Fluency Disord* 35: 141–145.

[66] Teichmann M; Dupoux E; Kouider S; Bachoud-Lévi AC (2006). The role of the striatum in processing language rules: evidence from word perception in Huntington's disease. *J Cogn Neurosci* 18(9):1555-69.

[67] Teichmann M; Gaura V; Démonet JF; Supiot F; Delliaux M; Verny C; Renou P; Remy P; Bachoud-Lévi AC (2008). Language processing within the striatum: evidence from a PET correlation study in Huntington's disease. *Brain* 131(Pt 4):1046-56.

[68] Teichmann M; Rosso C; Martini JB; Bloch I; Brugières P; Duffau H; Lehéricy S; Bachoud-Lévi AC (2015). A cortical-subcortical syntax pathway linking Broca's area and the striatum. *Hum Brain Mapp* 36:2270-2283.

[69] Tettamanti M; Moro A; Messa C; Moresco RM; Rizzo G; Carpinelli A; Matarrese M; Fazio F; Perani D (2005). Basal ganglia and language: phonology modulates dopaminergic release. *Neuroreport* 16: 397-401.

[70] Tomasi D; Volkow ND (2012). Resting functional connectivity of language networks: characterization and reproducibility. *Mol Psychiatry* 17(8):841-54.

[71] Wahl M; Marzinzik F; Friederici A D; Hahne A; Kupsch A; Schneider G H; Saddy D; Curio G; Klostermann F (2008). The human thalamus processes syntactic and semantic language violations. *Neuron* 59(5): 695–707.

[72] Whelan BM; Murdoch BE; Theodoros DG; Darnell R; Silburn P; Hall B (2004). Redefining functional models of basal ganglia organization: role for the posteroventral pallidum in linguistic processing? *Mov Disord* 19(11):1267-78.

[73] Zikopoulos B; Barbas H (2007). Circuits for multisensory integration and attentional modulation through the prefrontal cortex and the thalamic reticular nucleus in primates. *Rev Neurosci* 18: 417–438.

INDEX

C

D

E

F

G

H

N

O

P

Q

R

S

T

U

V

W

Y